Cheeseburgers for Seniors

—m—

*Top Ten Reasons Your Parents Don't Want to Move to Senior Living -
A Guide for Boomers and their Parents*

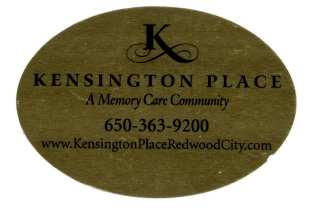

John D. Graham

Copyright © 2013 John D. Graham

All rights reserved.

ISBN-10: 0615873103
ISBN-13: 9780615873107

Preface

A Guide for Boomers & Parents

This handbook is meant to support those searching for care, seniors seeking to educate themselves on life options and families trying to understand the process. After twenty years of serving in executive leadership positions in senior services, I have developed an intimate understanding of the transitional process families experience when considering senior living. Too often, families are exhausted with no where to turn when they come across my path. Whether struggling with personal care, issues related to dementia or dealing with loss and grief, I have worked with hundreds of families who turned to us for support. While I have most recently served in executive leadership roles, I have always been "hands on". It has been a life mission for me, starting with my own father who died when I was nine. I can remember helping him wash his back with a sponge after his surgery for lung cancer. In those days, they made an incision from the sternum around to the back to remove the diseased portion of the lung. The stitches were spaced too far apart for my comfort, always concerned that too much pressure would damage the wound. I suppose life provided a direction and even a training program at nine years old in the small country bathroom with a curtain covering the water heater closet. Life is a symphony that ultimately harmonizes into a beautiful movement of meaning.

Over the years, I have stayed nights with dying loved ones after a full day of administrative work. Sleeping on the couch and listening intently to the labored breathing and the bubbling of the oxygen machine, sometimes presence is enough.

I have convinced a powerful community leader, far beyond my social class, to let me put on his shoes when impacted by dementia. Prominent men rarely find themselves having another man put on their shoes, much less losing their shoe to begin with. It is uncomfortable and unwelcome help when struggling to remember where you are. Necessity is the mother of invention. One day after observing this gentleman walking down the hall having lost one of his shoes, I picked up the shoe and tried to assist him to put it on. All to no avail. It finally dawned on me that I must play the shoe salesman to have my help received. Holding the loafer and presenting it to try for fit, I finally got my friend over to the bench with me. Kneeling down with the shoe, I asked him if he would like to try it on. He said yes. Our perceptions of me putting on his shoe were different. He was working with a salesperson to determine the right shoe. I was a caregiver struggling to find communication strategies to reach someone in another reality. In that moment, we found common ground to move through life together.

Helping caregivers to learn to redirect physical aggression from strong men twice their size, I once intervened in the "kidnapping" of a staff member when a resident decided he was leaving—one way or another. There is no training like experience.

Driving residents to church on Sunday, wondering what I would do if one of the ladies needed assistance in the restroom. Nothing substitutes for the human touch. Whether CEO or nurse or a kind parishioner on the bench beside you, the touch of love and compassion is help beyond measure.

In my early career, eighty was senior—even in senior living. After almost three decades in senior care, I am thrilled to say that eighty is not, by definition, old anymore. I have observed numerical age expand its limits. Ninety five is the new eighty.

I have also seen numerical age fade to the background of measurement, encountering ninety year olds who still snow ski. Getting old, in the mental, emotional and psychological sense has been pushed aside by many of the new courageous "aging pioneers" who have determined to age successfully. As much as care and compassion are a part of senior living, vibrancy and joy is equally a part. I have been on hayrides where the average age was eighty. I have watched nursing home residents who had difficulty walking, rowing a boat on a lake. Danced the two-step with Southern ladies who would never tell me their age but certainly twice that of mine. I have seen marriages for those above eighty, under the oak tree, after six weeks of courtship. I have also seen love triangles that almost came to blows. Time becomes more precious and the enlightened savor it and run headlong into love, never turning back. I have come to understand through shining examples that our fifty and forward years can be the most vibrant treasure of our time here on earth. As with all stages of life, it is what you make of it. The investment reaps the rewards.

While I am not an attorney, a doctor, a lawyer, a financial advisor or a geriatric social worker, I bring years of experience in supporting seniors and their families through life transitions related to the aging process. The primary purpose of the book is not to supplant the roles of experts who may be needed along the way but to educate, inform and engage people about decisions that can impact your most exciting stage of life.

No recent generations have had the luxury to look forward to the lifespan our generation will enjoy—what I call the third semester. The possibilities are limitless. My passion is to create awareness that we should look at our lives past fifty, not as categories or decades related to a certain age, but an entire bonus semester of thirty years to plan, execute and enjoy to the fullest. Create a life plan and sign up for the classes you love.

Remember your twenties when completing your education? Finances, housing and careers dominated your life concerns. With the uncertainty came excitement, dreams and plans with endless possibilities. With decades of life experience and the security of now knowing our capabilities, the last thing we should do is sit back and wait for life to happen. It is a time to grab life by the horns and revel in it like a puppy in a field of clover.

Let me disclose up front, I am a rabid enthusiast for older people. I have loved the company of those fifty and above since childhood. Over the course of life, I have often chosen the company of seniors over my peers. Unfortunately, there are many stereotypes that have developed about aging. I have not found these to be valid. Sometimes, I find that stereotypes enable us to pigeonhole people who don't behave as we expect them to and affiliate this behavior with age. People say that older people don't like change. People categorize older people as stubborn. More often than not, I find behaviors related to aging stereotypes, to be completely normal for anyone else in the same circumstance, regardless of age.

Consider someone who does not want to move to a nursing home. Do you want to move to a two hundred square foot room with people coming in and out of your private space at all hours of the day or night? How would you like to have one closet, no microwave and one window at your house? Eat food from the same restaurant, three times per day, 365 days a year for the rest of your life? Does your answer to these questions make you stubborn? Resistant to change? Or just a grownup who knows what they prefer?

Consider the memory impaired senior with low vision who refuses to take a bath with assistance. This person may not remember nurses or their own daughter from day to day or minute to minute. Someone, whom they do not know, walks into their private living space and promptly instructs them that they will be taking their clothes off and giving them a bath. Someone else they did not know just came through and rifled through their chest of drawers taking their clothes. They refuse to have someone they do not remember force them into the bathroom and strip their clothes off. Is this "inappropriate or combative behavior"? Absolutely not. It is completely logical and appropriate behavior given the situation with the information and cognition available. You would not allow someone you do not know to come into your private space, take your clothes and then get naked in front of them in the bathroom.

Conversely, if someone comes into your room, bends down to eye level, makes an introduction and communicates clearly that they are a nurse here to help you, pointing to their name badge, you might be more open to receiving assistance with a bath. A smile and some familiar conversation using your name and mentioning getting dressed before your daughter comes to visit, might warm you up even more to the idea of a bath. Empathy with you about the pain and stiffness in your hip, offering to help you so that it doesn't hurt so much to get into the shower, might help. A big fluffy spa robe to keep you warm before you get into the shower, some beautifully scented lotion and a nice cup of tea to enjoy when you finish with the shower, might win you over to the idea completely.

Stereotypes develop when we interpret behavior as consistent with a category of people and inconsistent with our own behavior. Empathy and understanding go a long way to explode stereotypes.

While at fifty, you may not consider a warm shower, a fluffy robe, compassionate care and a nice cup of tea on a winter day, high on your list of quality of life measures, your opinion could change as you age. You are not always thirsty when you start a bike ride, but a bottle of water can be just what the doctor ordered after several miles up and down a few hills. Orchestrating our quality of life for every stage of aging drastically improves the chances that what you treasure most will be yours when you need it.

In our prior discussion about nursing homes, I questioned if we might enjoy moving to one. As we age, and at the appropriate time, having someone coming in and out of our private space and available twenty four hours per day can provide a feeling of security and nurture. Having to look only to one closet with clothes that are easy to fasten and comfortable can become a blessing. Not having a microwave but having someone bring you a snack at beck and call may become more appealing. If our joints ache, walking to the bathroom ten feet away in a small room may prevent the fear of an incontinence episode on the way there. Hand rails to stand up from the toilet may give us a sense of security and control. The point is we may value different lifestyles at different stages of life but only *we* can decide what we value!

What I have found to be true is that healthy aging is a frontier to be explored. My goal is to convince you to be proactive and take charge of your own destiny. An educated consumer is an empowered consumer.

I founded my company, LifeSwell, with a mission committed to "Inspiring Crescendos for Life-Fifty and Forward". Now more than ever, fifty is just the beginning! As you read the book, I hope to increase your gratitude for the choices your life investments have created, the family you love and inspire you to actively engage in the opportunities they provide. At LifeSwell, we provide assistance with senior living options and lifestyle transitions. Whether struggling with a mid-life employment transition, considering long-term care financing, senior living, downsizing/relocation options or family dynamics, we are here for you. We provide private coaching and educational and motivational speaking on topics relevant to those fifty and forward. You may contact me for more information at LifeSwell50@gmail.com or telephone at 818.578.8917.

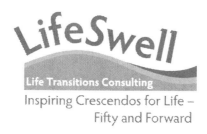

Contents

Preface	iii
1. The Unique Generation	1
2. Family Dynamics for Boomers	7
3. Considerations for Parents	21
4. Trends in Senior Housing Choices	39
5. Cheeseburgers for Seniors	43
a. Reason #1: The Food Is Not Good!	44
6. Operations and Safety Considerations	65
a. Reason #2: It Smells Bad!	65
7. Profit vs. Nonprofit Communities	75
8. Lifestyle and Care	81
a. Reason #3: I Don't Want to Live around Those "Old People!"	83

9. Parents Are People Too!   91

    a. Reason #4: I'll Cross That Bridge When I Get to It. Gladys and I Have Each Other. We Don't Need a Retirement Community.   93

10. Senior Living Options   105

11. Incorrect Assumptions Steal Your Potential   121

    a. Reason #5: I Don't Like Bingo!   121

12. Financial Considerations   129

    a. Reason #6: I Can't Afford It!   129

13. Regulation   141

14. Stereotypes May Isolate You   147

    a. Reason #7: Real Men Don't Live in Those Places.   147

    b. Reason #8: I'm Gay/Lesbian/Bisexual/Transgendered. I Wouldn't Fit in There.   150

    c. Reason #9: I'm a Loner. I Don't Want to Be Around All Those People!   152

15. Stuff, Stuff, and More Stuff…   155

    a. Reason #10: The Apartments Are Too Small! I Need Space for My Stuff!   155

16. The Final Pitch   161

I
The Unique Generation

This book is written for boomers and their parents. Whether you were born in early 1960's and on the younger end of boomerhood or you are eighty and considering your own needs, this book is for you. The transitions we experience in older adulthood are some of the most monumental we ever encounter.

We are a unique generation. Our parents will live longer and stronger than any generation before them. Boomers have a third semester of life spanning thirty years to thrive and enjoy. This is a new family dynamic. Today we have the ninety-two-year-old mother driving her seventy-two-year-old son to physical therapy while the son's fifty-year-old daughter helps with some aspects of both their lives. Who would have thought we would see three generations in AARP safe driving school? This may be a photo opportunity for one of those multiple-generation photos for the family album. Only no babies are required for these three generations.

I approach some topics with humor. Please take my banter in the spirit in which it was intended. People who are fifty-plus—parents or children—are not feeble. We still have a sense of humor. We all know we are getting older, and approaching the aging process with some fun certainly makes it easier. We are not too fragile to take a joke. We would rather not be perceived as some protected class because we have lived to see fifty. Most of us plan to impact our culture and the lives of those around us in the best way possible. Aging is not always easy, and a laugh or two along the way makes it much more interesting.

The Sandwich Generation

Today, families are more geographically dispersed than ever. Boomer children have pursued careers that require relocation. Grandchildren are involved in more academic, athletic and social pursuits than any generation before them. In an effort to give our children better teenage years than we had, we say yes to soccer, debate club, excursions, sports and a variety of other time intensive activities that were neither available nor economically feasible when we were teenagers. Our children do not have part-time jobs as we did, which places higher demands on family finances driving us farther and farther into maximizing our incomes and prioritizing work above family. Our consumerist culture places high value on providing our children the next smart phone, designer clothes and automobiles needed to assuage the intense peer pressure. Being a parent is a challenge in today's world. Parenting can greatly impact the time and energy we have left for being the adult child of your now aging parent. I understand that it is indeed challenging to spend time with your parents. I argue that it is an investment of time that you will never regret, keeping in mind that you cannot do it all.

If we see our parents sporadically, visual cues to their well-being may escape us entirely. We only see them several times a year for a limited time. We don't notice that additional locks have been added to doors. The car has a few more dings where mom or dad hit the curb at the grocery store. We may not know that they are no longer driving at night and experiencing social isolation from friends and community. You may not see the cupboards bare of food due to the recent frenzied shopping for a large load of groceries to prepare Thanksgiving Dinner.

Seniors may have values that some consider "outdated thinking" but the jury is still out. Our culture has abandoned some long held and successful intergenerational approaches to life, due to the demands of the modern world. My guess is that much of the wisdom of our parents will increase in value as we relate to our own children in the aging dynamic. Most parents want their families nearby geographically and put great value on the closeness of relationships. We see this manifest in ideas like calling your mom every week. Coming home for five days during the holidays. Planning destination vacations to include as many family members as we can.

With our busy lives, we can sometimes see this as an obligation to be met. The logistics of airline tickets, rental cars, the teenage daughter who needs three suitcases and allocating the time out to be with our families, can seem daunting. The desire to spend time expressed by our older relatives can seem less than pragmatic. You think "if mom only knew my schedule for the holiday season." Or "I haven't had a real vacation in three years. I'd rather go on a vacation." Sadly, we don't stop to realize that this life opportunity is one that will not always be there.

We can create opposition thinking in our mind categorizing family time as just another stressor to be dealt with in my already hectic life. We may even interpret requests for family time as selfish on the part of our parents or grow resentful when they will not travel to your location to visit. We are so busy. It would be so much easier if they would just come to visit us.

Challenges Older Adults Face

As we age, there are multiple factors that make travel difficult for older adults. Mobility, medical conditions, bodily functions, caregiving for their spouse, depression and a host of other life impacts does not make for a level playing field in the travel category. We do not know that mom is wearing incontinence products. Dad cannot hear as well as he used to and the airport noises fill him with anxiety. Mom is having some memory loss and can no longer drive to the grocery store. Dad is increasingly becoming a caregiver for mom and he is exhausted. Not to mention, concerned about how well she will travel. They may not be accustomed to airport security procedures of today and dread the process, having heard multiple horror stories about it in the media. Between mom and dad, they may have fifteen prescriptions for which refill dates are staggered and must be obtained for a trip. Some medications require blood monitoring, full meals to take the medications and side effects such as dizziness or frequent urination. Parents may feel vulnerable in locations where urgent medical care is not covered by their health plan. I write this segment not to stereotype older adults as frail, isolated or incapable, but to set forth some variables that require understanding on the part of the adult child.

Parents do not want to appear needy or dependent. Sometimes the amount of time spent with family is so limited parents do not want to engage in conversations about aging issues. Appropriately, they have a right to privacy and dignity just as anyone else. We have to remember that being an aging parent is new for them as well. They have always supported you as their children, not the reverse. We hear many parents say "we don't want to be a burden to our children". Discussing aging issues can be an uncomfortable conversation that may equate to feelings of dependence or shame about loss of control over one's life. Not discussing these situations, can also be a protection strategy if they fear being forced out of their homes into another living situation. Dad may be covering for mom's memory loss because he fears that they will be separated and his role as caregiver will be supplanted.

Time to Evolve

The family dynamic between parent and adult child must evolve for continued enjoyment of the relationship. How many times have we heard someone say "old people become children again"? While this statement may allow for compartmentalizing behaviors that are unfamiliar to us in other adults, it is neither correct nor a dignified approach to an older person. Some conditions related to aging may have similarities to child-like behavior, but when investigated further, it is not an appropriate comparison. A sure fire way to sabotage a genuine relationship with seniors is to internalize this notion and behave as if it were true. While you may need to provide support for your parents, empathy is probably the most valuable tool in these relationships. Understanding what is happening is far more important than having a solution for every challenge. You cannot become the parent and you will not be able to guide all decisions to a perfect outcome. If you leave paternalistic thinking toward your parents, here and now, you will alleviate relationship challenges and corresponding guilt later on. You only need walk beside them and support them.

Spending quality time in conversation leads to understanding what support they need or want. Options to address aging challenges are varied and fluid. Engaging in productive conversations with your parents about their challenges, their desire for support and their plans for addressing these challenges is the first step. It has to be their plan, their options—not yours. It is appropriate for you to educate yourself on options. Support their discovery process but leave control in their court unless safety becomes an issue. You never want to communicate that you are "going to put them in a home" or "you will have to this if that happens." They are adults and you really don't have the right. They will hesitate to be honest with you about their challenges if they feel it is going to lead to their loss of control. I emphasize to you supporting the principles of choice and self-determination for your parents. These two foundational principles will pave the way for a smoother journey.

In past generations, it has been rare to see individuals in three generations of a family all over fifty years old. It is a life pattern our generation will pioneer. With the challenges and complexity of health care, educating and supporting one another is crucial to successful relationships throughout the aging process. While your daughter may not remember which smart phone model she had when she was fourteen, she will cherish shared time and memories passed on from your parents. Shared traditions and family legacy is a gift beyond value. Remember, the pattern you role model for your children with your parents will impact the way you are treated when you are eighty and they are fifty.

II

Family Dynamics for Boomers

How do children behave after fifty? In many cases, much as they always have. Mean girls are still mean girls. Jocks are still jocks. The parent/child dynamic can be baffling, both to us and to those who observe us. Healthy aging involves an evolution in the parent/child dynamic. Daddy can no longer fix everything. Mom may not want to make holiday meals for fifty. Neither may have time to babysit your grandchildren. Not to mention, grandchildren may be thirty and need a place to live, not to be babysat. Although they are seventy-plus, your parents may never need or want your help. Please don't view this as rejection. As we have discussed, the old adage that "old people become like children again" is neither a true nor a respectful statement. It is demeaning and paternalistic to identify people as child-like because they need help. Conversely, you do not become the parent if you provide help. People of all ages help each other every day in varied ways with varying outcomes and we don't label them children.

Children-Now-Adults

There is a continuum of behavior with adult children. I label these polar opposites as *children-now-adults* or *now-adult-children*. Notice the word children placed first in a category where adults continue to see their parents only as parents. *Children-now-adults* can never imagine their parents needing help or including them in conversations on life choices. Children-now-adults may expect advice, financial support, and a variety of other grown-up services from their parents, but they do not engage in a two-way adult relationship. They look to their parents only as parents. At this end of the continuum, you may find passivity, denial, dependence, disorientation, self-centeredness, and a break down in these children-now-adults during difficult life transitions with their parents. These adults still see themselves as children and can feel lost when parents are no longer willing or able to play the parental role in ways that were functional in earlier life. This mode of interrelation can rob adult children of the opportunity to truly know and love their parents as individuals who are fascinating and exceptional people apart from the parental role. Don't miss getting to know a great friend just because they happen to be your parent!

Now-Adult-Children

Now-adult-children may feel a responsibility to "take care" of their parents. Bossy children may assume this paternalistic role at the drop of a hat, giving advice, making decisions, and imposing their expectations on their parents. These behaviors can stem from a feeling of responsibility, love, or compassion. Their approach may be to interfere with their parents' freedom of choice and self-determination. Given past family dynamics with aging generations, they may buy into the idea that older people become children again and that now they are to be the parents. Their behaviors may be well intentioned, but hasty. Moving your mom halfway across the country into your own home when she is only seventy-five and doing her own thing is riddled with consequences that cannot be reversed easily. At this end of the continuum, you may find aggressiveness, assumption of life choices, dominance, pressure, control, and emotionally reactive decisions. Now-adult-children may manipulate with guilt or paternalism. This approach is the quickest route to conflict with parents and ultimately isolation of the demanding child. This approach may internalize undue responsibility and corresponding guilt, characterized by the saying, "If I don't take care of Mom, who will?" The answer is—someone else will. When we place unrealistic expectations on ourselves, it can ultimately lead to a physical or mental state that renders us UNABLE to play the role. Should this happen, one learns the hard way that if we cannot—someone else will.

Understand that polar opposite ends of the adult child behavior continuum rarely exist. Use this concept to determine where you are today. It can help with self-awareness and appropriate responses as transitions come.

Hopefully, quite a few life markers will occur before you find your family in a caregiving situation. Your approach to these events can drastically impact the journey if a caregiving relationship develops.

Taking Care of Yourself

If you are currently a caregiver, you may feel that you are a long distance down a difficult road and there is little room for corrective navigation. The consequences and options for decision-making related to aging can be overwhelming. If these decisions have been neglected or denied, you may find yourself feeling ill-prepared and out of control.

Affirm yourself. Realize that your concern, empathy and compassion may be enough. The level at which you have expected yourself to assist may be unrealistic for you or any other human being. Find peace within yourself. Peace to do only what you are able. Peace to set boundaries for what you will and can do without harming your own well-being. In seeking to help others, if you expend yourself in the process, your capacity to help may be diminished. Whether you believe in a mainstream view of God or some other mode of spirituality, know that your spiritual being comes first. Within your spirit lies a healthy way to approach your challenges. You are not responsible for any crisis that may have arisen due to your parent's procrastination, denial, or passivity in prior decision-making. Accepting these consequences without discussion can lead to guilt, resentment, and a personal sense of inadequacy.

If this book finds you in crisis and uncertain as to where to turn, know that it will be all right. There are days when we find ourselves not knowing what tomorrow will bring or how we will manage ourselves, much less support someone else. It's OK. Know now that you must support yourself first. In order to give, you must be given to. Sometimes we can only receive from God the care we allow ourselves. You cannot be everything to someone. I frequently see the caregivers and nurturers among us, spent and hopeless because they have given more than life has replenished. Only you can reverse this pattern. You must allow for self-care in order to give back in meaningful ways.

You may be a son or daughter who has taken on care for your parents. We often tell ourselves we alone are responsible. This can never be. If you were absent, where then would the responsibility lie? Life moves forward whether we are crumbling along the way or moving along, productively using the energy we have to give. You alone can never take the guilt for consequences of a decision you were neither engaged nor empowered to make. Ultimately, we can only come alongside one another. Only with personal strength can we contribute. If you are exhausted, replenish. If you are done, you must be done. If you have the strength, reach out for help. If you do not, sit alone and rest in silence until your way becomes clear again. God does not ask that we destroy ourselves to be there for another.

As passionately as I want to help you understand the senior living journey, I want to also caution you about pacing yourself for the trip. Physical conditions such as fibromyalgia have been connected to caregiver stress. Poor nutrition, poor sleep and physical exhaustion is a reality that affects caregivers who have unrealistic expectations of themselves.

Where Do I Turn?

You may need to reach out for help.

- Your local chapter of the **Alzheimer's Association** may provide educational referral, and support services if you are caring for someone with cognitive impairment. Locate your chapter at www.alz.org

- Local **Councils on Aging** provide referral services and often supportive care such as Meals on Wheels. The website of the National Association of Area Agencies on Aging (www.n4a.org) provides an elder care locator service under "Programs" tab. This site has a wealth of information on issues related to aging.

- For information on Medicare HMO supplements and insurance issues, see www.seniorresourceguide.com/directories/National/SHIP to get a listing for your state Senior Health Insurance Information Program (SHIIP)

- The official Medicare site (www.medicare.gov) provides a wealth of information on Medicare programs and services.

- ***Social workers*** in hospitals can educate you on options for after-care should your loved one be hospitalized.

- ***Certified Geriatric Care Managers*** can be located through www.caremanager.org. This is the National Association of Professional Geriatric Care Managers.

- ***Physicians*** are often aware of good programs where their patients have found quality services.

- ***Charitable organizations*** such as Volunteers of America provide a wide range of senior services.

- *Faith-based organizations,* such as Catholic Charities, have programs to support seniors and their families.

- ***Adult day care centers*** can be located through the National Adult Day Services Association at www.nadsa.org

- ***Leading Age*** is a national association of non-profit senior services providers with over 6,000 members. www.leadingage.org provides location services, consumer education and advocacy on a variety of senior health issues

If financial resources are available, there are certified geriatric care managers (listed above) such as nurses or social workers who can help you navigate the journey for an hourly fee. Don't get these confused with agencies that refer seniors to residential or care options in return for a "finder's fee" for placement. I am not making a judgment about their services. Just know that these agencies get paid a fee when you move to a senior living community. There is a vested interest in placement in a residential setting. These agencies may be well-versed in the range of options available in your area. They can match you with services that fit your budget. They can help to educate you about the quality and range of services you can expect to receive from senior living providers.

Getting Help from Other Family Members

Family members are often willing to help. It is rare these days to find a family where someone has not grappled with retirement choices. Ask for advice and education from those who have addressed the issue within their own families. If you are geographically distant, start a dialogue with family members who are located nearer your parent for resources and support networks. Conversely, if you are distant and partnering with a brother or sister who is local in caring for your parents, realize that you cannot understand unless you are nearby. It may be hard for you to understand why your parent has given up driving if you haven't been called by the supermarket manager when your loved one cannot locate the car and make his or her way home. You may not see the sticky notes on the fridge reminding your mom to pay the utility bill or the chair relocated to the bath to provide stabilization for getting in and out of the shower.

As children, we need to understand how to support each other. Realize first that you *must* support each other. Uninformed advice can lead to guilt and frustration on the part of the primary caregiver. Family members have a vast array of perceptions of what others expect, which can lead to frustration and anger. While your sibling may be listening to your helpful "advice" from two states away, he or she may not have the time or energy to explain why your scenario is not workable. Your sibling may also feel a sense of intense pressure to live up to your expectations. That sibling's commitment to doing the best thing for your mom and dad could leave him or her feeling hopeless and alone. Advice with no assistance will eventually lead to a breakdown in the relationship. Don't be an armchair quarterback without an appropriate level of empathy.

Dealing with Denial

As the child of an aging parent, you may find it difficult to be objective. Denial is often a safe place to retreat. Seeing your dad struggle to get out of the passenger side of the car doesn't always alert you to the reality of aging. Changes in ability can happen quickly with aging. You must strive to be realistic about challenges along the way. It is also important to remember that your parents are adults. They have the right to make decisions that may be ill-advised. Until these decisions indicate an unsafe environment or serious cognitive impairment, you may not have the right to involve yourself in parental decisions without invitation.

Conditions That Require Communication

If cognitive decline is evident, geriatric psychiatry programs can help with assessments and baseline data on the functioning level of your parent. This process can empower you and your parent with tools to address the need. Assessment can alleviate the unspoken fear that mom has Alzheimer's, when memory deficits may be related to other issues. A baseline assessment repeated at periodic intervals will give both you and your loved ones a measurement tool to identify when things are remaining the same cognitively or medications or treatment may be needed.

Cognitive impairments can be related to light strokes in the brain, sometimes called TIAs. Severe cognitive impairments can result when seniors undergo anesthesia for a procedure. It can take days or weeks for the effect of anesthesia to subside. Urinary tract infections and corresponding dehydration can mirror cognitive impairments. Parkinson's related dementia can appear differently than other forms of dementia. Realize that "dementia" is a symptom, not a disease. It can be caused by a number of health conditions.

Depression is prevalent in the aging community and often undiagnosed. Older seniors may view a psychiatric condition as a stigma. Untreated depression can start a spiral of numerous challenges that could be avoided with proper diagnosis and treatment. Seniors of our generation may be more comfortable approaching depression with a private therapist or social worker before pursuing an appointment with a psychiatrist. LCSWs (licensed clinical social workers) are a treasure of compassion and support who can establish trust and eventually work through resistance to medical treatment if needed. They often work with psychiatrists who prescribe and monitor the drug interventions while your parent remains in therapy with the social worker.

Fear leads to denial and resistance in pursuing help that may be needed. I have found that unspoken fears can be the greatest barrier to getting help that can drastically improve quality of life. When you think about life events related to aging, one can understand why depression is prevalent. Losing friends or family members to death repeatedly can impact one who has limited coping skills for multiple tragic experiences. Heck, you can have the best coping skills in the world and it is only human to have challenges when you have lost important people in your life.

Life Example - I have seen families struggle for months or years, unaware of resources, throw up their hands in surrender. I once moved a gentleman into a senior community I oversaw. This man had experienced multiple auto accidents and dangerous situations due to his progressing Parkinson's disease. His children finally took him out to their family farm and left him with no car, only a golf cart. Of course, they constantly checked on him and brought him groceries and the like. The farm stimulated his most internalized programmed memory pattern for daily life. He survived at the farm for a time, most likely undernourished and disoriented on many fronts. He vehemently refused assistance, and his children didn't know what else to do. He was an intimidating, dominant personality, and his bouts of behavior issues did not calm the interaction one bit. They were still respectful of his parental authority to the point of neglect. Unfortunately, he eventually ended up on a major interstate highway in his golf cart, delusional and confused. Not a good outcome.

My goal is to give you information and proactive strategies while respecting your parents' choices to avoid these crisis scenarios.

Promises You May Not Be Able to Make

How many times have I heard a daughter, weeping, say, "I promised Mom I would not put her in a home". What a promise! It is like promising your ten-year-old son who plays sports that you will never take him to an emergency room. If he breaks a bone or gets hit in the head with a ball, are you really able to keep a promise like that? Think about the dynamics of promising *not* to do something that may ultimately save your parents' lives or make their lives easier and better. It is a difficult spot to be in. If your parents ask you to promise not to put them in a home, it is only fair that you be able to return with, "Should you need care, what would you have me do, and where would you like to receive it? Tell me your plan."

This is an exceptional starting point for a conversation that can be truthful and productive. Unrealistic promises reinforce denial on the part of your parents and leave you holding the ball in a no-win scenario. Engage your parents in a discovery process to identify options they consider acceptable. A collaborative discovery process is not you going out and gathering brochures and information to bring home for their review. The list of acceptable options starts with their input. It continues with an agreement that choice and self-determination can only be accomplished with their involvement. Once gathered, outline the resources available and how they are to be used. We would never engage a child in such a process. It is different with parents. They are adults and have earned the dignity of choice. They have not, however, earned the right to put you in a situation where you have to figure out what is acceptable if they have eliminated the most plausible option. It is their responsibility to tell you—*if not this, then what?*

If fear and denial have prevented your parents from making plans for their own care, you may find yourself in a crisis or need-driven scenario. The worst part of a need-driven move to senior living is the "putting" of someone somewhere. Putting someone somewhere indicates a loss of control for your parent(s) and possibly an undesirable outcome. It makes someone the bad guy if it doesn't turn out well. Think about instances in your own life where someone made a choice for you. While "Mom made me take piano lessons" is stellar if you end up performing at Carnegie Hall, you might not talk about your piano lessons with the same tone if you lose out on a baseball scholarship and blame your mom because of it. The same goes for senior living. Choices—and specifically delayed choices—can have impactful outcomes.

Avoidance and Denial

While many people avoid considering senior living, these living arrangements can be beautiful places filled with life and love. Senior living can bring new life to a person who has lost a spouse and lived an isolated existence for many years. Sharing the experiences of your peers can alleviate anxiety caused by issues related to aging. Knowing someone who successfully faced a challenge can provide courage and empowerment to walk a difficult path. People flower and life becomes new again. As an adult child, you can do the research, help with the cost, and find the best choice only to hear Mom or Dad say, "I am not going to one of those places." When you get right down to it, this is the most difficult part of the process. Months, sometimes years, of research, visits, and educating yourself about the choices end with an impasse. Your best resource in this scenario is a peer for your parents who has made a successful transition to senior living. Most senior living communities will make a connection for you. They will identify a resident to meet with your parent(s) and discuss the transition.

As the dialogue continues and your parents identify their priorities, they often discover that the "old folks" in a community of their choosing are not so different from themselves, and then the idea of a communal setting seems far less abhorrent. After attending a Pilates class for seniors, traveling to Spain on a cruise with community residents, or lunching with a colleague who continues to work from retirement, senior living might not seem so distasteful. The key is agreement on self-determination, communication, and increasing familiarity with the options available. Self-determination is best accomplished from a well-informed platform.

Left Holding the Bag

If you are left with the responsibility of the decision, chances are, denial or fear has put you into the driver's seat. Driving someone to the dentist is not always appreciated, even though years of avoiding dental care might make it necessary. Don't be surprised if your assistance is not always lauded. Through this journey, remember these themes:

- Ask questions about desired outcomes without influencing the answer.

- Trust your gut.

- Value choice and self-determination for your parents.

- Don't internalize fear and anxiety on the part of your parent as a lack of appreciation for your help.

Chances are the avoidance has been long-standing.

"I Am Not Going to One of Those Places"

Statements like the one above hurt and leave you bewildered about what to do next, especially if your search is need-driven. When a health concern arises that cannot be managed at home, you are left sitting in the seat of responsibility. We are often ill-equipped in many ways to play the role. It requires tenacity and the willingness to educate oneself on the options available. It requires emotional maturity in a relationship where you have traditionally been the follower, not the leader. The dynamic can be unsettling. Your parents have always known the answer. Always led the way. And now, as an adult child, you experience your parents exhibiting denial, emotional reactions, and a resistance to making a life transition. It leaves you feeling responsible and sometimes helpless in a situation where your concern for the safety and well-being of your parent is not good enough nor appreciated.

"To one of those places…" indicates that you are trying to move them into a prison, work camp, or worse. The tone says it all. Unfortunately, sometimes the tone is justified. Not every senior community is created equal. Based on the choices your parents have or their perception of senior living, it may feel, to them, like a death sentence. If you have never walked into a nursing home and been greeted immediately by the stench of urine and the sight of thirty overmedicated residents slumped over in a circle in their wheelchairs—take a tour of one.

Medicare provides a star rating system that gives you minimal guidance, based on regulatory surveys, as to the quality of a nursing home. The maximum star level is five. Few attain this level, but if the star level is two or less, chances are you will have some experiences on your tour that will help you understand the fear in your parents' tone and not take it personally. (www.medicare.gov) Even with the best nursing home choice, life changes. Imagine living in a room lit by fluorescent lights with care staff entering and exiting at all times of the day or night. A drastic lifestyle change to say the least. Perception of senior living may be based on bad experiences. Possibly a visit to a friend or a horror story of someone else's family member has colored their thinking. In this book, I hope to give you tools, information, and reinforcement to ease the difficulty of the journey. There are great nursing homes, great senior living communities, and great people caring for elders. You just have to find them.

I understand this situation from both sides. Having been a senior-living industry professional for over twenty years, I see the conversation play out over and over again with wounded emotions, regret, and guilt beyond measure. Working with family members, who are often struggling with their own life challenges, and genuinely wanting to help your parents can feel unmanageable. Your parents took care of you, and you certainly have a commitment to do your best by them.

Few people are sufficiently educated regarding the different retirement offerings to assist from a knowledgeable perspective. It could take months just to get up to speed on what's out there, what is best for your parents, and what is acceptable to them. The healthcare category includes Medicare, Medicare HMO's, prescription drug benefits and ancillary health care policies that supplement Medicare benefits. There are financial issues, long-term care insurance, reverse mortgages, and a host of other issues related to aging. Time to do the research in every category is often in short supply. When a crisis necessitates immediate decisions, you must enlist resources such as the ones discussed earlier. A call to a professional who deals with these issues frequently can be a far better investment of time and energy than weeks of research on your part.

III

Considerations for Parents

Let's talk about the language of "putting one somewhere." This is the opposite of *choice* and *self-determination*, two recurring themes in this book. Being put somewhere is the scenario you have the power to avoid! Putting someone somewhere indicates a loss of control or choice by the "puttee." A scenario where your loved one has to make the choice for you is the one you want to avoid.

As a parent, you have a duty to inform yourself and make your own choices if you value self-determination. In most cases, children only step in and make important life choices for their parents when parents are in denial or avoiding making their own choices. With this situation, it is common for feelings of paternalism to surface between child and parent. "I know what's best for you," might be the child's unspoken message. "I have done all the research." "This is what I think you need to do." "Why are you making this so difficult?"

If hearing these types of messages from your adult children in reference to your need for care makes you feel uneasy, form your intentions now so you can take preventative measures to avoid these conversations. Your children cannot know what it feels like to leave the neighborhood where your life's dream was built. They cannot yet understand what it is like to lose half your friends within five years.

In my experience, choice and self-determination are the lifeblood of remaining active, vibrant, and hopeful as one ages. When hope dies, people die. While physical capacity may change with age, the choice of what you have for dinner, what music you will hear, and how you will get where you want to go are huge quality-of-life issues. If you have ever had a friend who chose to give up driving or, worse yet, had someone take his or her keys away, you know how this blow to independence can have a drastic impact on your outlook. Maybe you only go to the grocery store and play bridge during a week, but the autonomy to do either, or choose not to, is something many of us take for granted. You have the power to control your destiny. Denial won't get you there.

Get Excited

With focus and intention, retirement can provide the most enjoyable decades of life. As a generation, we have been able to do and have more. More houses. More work choices. More convenience. Better education. More vacations. More control of all the things that affect our lives. And now, yet another bonus: more years of life itself. What greater blessing could one imagine? To whom much is given, much is expected. Expect more of yourself in regards to this blessing you have been given. Don't allow the choices for self-fulfillment to slip away by failing to make a plan. Hiding your head in the sand and letting aging happen to you is not a good strategy.

Start by reigniting your passions. Review your list of enjoyable and fulfilling visions of your retirement. For starters, prioritize these and enumerate them by cost, number of years you would like to pursue, and location (if related to travel or a second home you are maintaining).

Your Passions

We can expect some decrease in agility and mobility as life goes on. You might choose your sixth decade as your golfing and whitewater rafting decade and save art history and yoga for your eighth decade. This doesn't mean that the two are mutually exclusive. Just realize that time and resources are limited. If you have your plan mapped out, you can allocate both passions to the times when you can best enjoy them. Activities such as exercise, Pilates, and yoga can have far-reaching effects on how well you live your future years. As we age, balance is not a skill we use as frequently as in prior years. Balance achieved through exercise can be a key factor in maintaining mobility and preventing a debilitating fall.

Come Up with a Timeframe

Plan for the stages of your retirement. List life events that trigger choices you will have made in advance. If I can no longer drive… If my cognitive function declines… f my friends move away… If my partner dies… Choose those triggers that impact your quality of life, corresponding decisions to be made and work backward. Some examples…

- If I have two hospitalizations in a twelve month period, we will leave the lake house and move nearer medical services.

- If my mini-mental cognitive score decreases below 24, I will not continue to live alone. I will move to XYZ independent living retirement option.

If female family members all live to ninety and beyond, choose ninety as your target date and move backward. If you get more years, then you will have another gratitude opportunity. If one of your parents lived to be eighty-four and you are now seventy, you may want to break your plan up into three- or five-year increments instead of decades. The point is to realize that you could have another lifetime to experience. Plan it well!

If you love your home and see owning it as an asset, determine a timeframe that you would like to stay in your home. It could be to pay off the mortgage, liquidate the asset, and then embark on your travel decade. It could be until your grandchildren or great-grandchildren graduate from their respective universities and move away. List the expenses you incur with taxes, insurance, home maintenance, repairs, and utilities. Have a finite idea of what the cost of keeping your home represents. Consider the advantages of liquidating your home and investing the money. Over thirty years, an alternative strategy could add considerably to your financial quality of life. Whether you choose a continuing care retirement community (CCRC), an active adult community, or a downsized life in a condo, your housing outlay could be considerably less. It could be more, but include the added values of life care services, safety, or quality social environments. Engaging your financial advisor in these discussions can be a valuable resource in creating your plan.

One or Multiple Moves?

Joining a CCRC will allow you to relocate once and move within the same campus as you need care or services. Downsizing to a condo may require relocation to assisted living and then later to a nursing home if medical care is needed. Bringing care into your condo is also a choice but can isolate you from outside relationships. The friends you make at a CCRC will often provide you with a continuing group of friends as some of you move together to higher levels of care.

You will need to weigh the value of the cost of maintaining your home in relation to other things you would like to do now or at a later stage of life. While it is true that life expectancy has increased, keep in mind that your target dates have uncontrolled variables, such as your own or your partner's health issues. Delaying choices can drastically impact the time you have to live each passion fully.

You may add up your home expense budget and decide you want to downsize in six months. If you have a passion you are working toward, this is easily doable. Yes, I have seen singles and couples downsize in as little as three months!

Deciding to Downsize

There are moving and home organization services that assist you with going through your possessions, keeping the ones you want, and divesting the rest. You can locate them easily. Their names often contain the word "transitions." These companies will outline what they can do for you. They often have organizing, moving, and even estate sale services. The focus of their business is usually downsizing seniors to assisted living communities. Don't let this scare you! In my move from Louisiana to Los Angeles, I engaged such a company to pack and transport my items to California. When they arrived, I hired a Los Angeles branch of the franchise to unpack and place my things. It was the best move I ever made, and I wasn't even fifty then! Senior moving services are yet another resource with repeated experience in life choices that you may only make once.

The proceeds from estate sales can generate funds to enhance your travel stage or enable you to purchase better finishes and amenities in your new residence. For those fortunate enough to have lived through the midcentury modern era (1948–1970), you may have home furnishings that are worth more than your car! Within your life plan, you can list having appraisals for items that may have increased in value and use these proceeds for a specific purpose.

Your family may be included in the process and given the responsibility of moving the items they would like to have. If everyone wants everything, label what you are giving up with numbers. Have a family dinner and let your "qualified" progeny draw numbers out of a hat for their desired items. Heck, I would even charge an admission price to be donated to your favorite charity! Certainly worth it if there is a grand piano in the mix. It might even finance the art classes you are planning to take.

In making this endeavor fun and rewarding, you could also attach a small price to items, with the proceeds to be donated to the charity of choice. You may group several items together that relate to a story or family outing as a memory box. Think of it as scrapbooking in three dimensions!

A lifetime of memories can be recycled to give something back. This approach gives you a positive perspective. That orange leather chair of ours from 1965 turned out to be a midcentury jewel, and we donated the proceeds to our great-grandson's nonprofit grade school to support programs for autistic children. Your life treasures and accumulations can have the power to give you joy in leveraging them to make life better for someone else or creating a legacy for generations to come. Don't look at divestiture as an ending, but as a giving.

By the way, if you have a grand piano, this takes a load off your plate. Moving a piano adds considerable weight to the moving quote. If no one wants the grand piano, you can make some cash on the sale. Buy a new keyboard with sound effects and recording capability for your new music composition stage of life. Your future may be sitting in the living room you dust twice a week that no one ever sits in. Look at your life in terms of the assets it has afforded you. Whether it is furniture you don't use anymore or experience that allows you to teach an art class, open your eyes to the jewels that are in your life chest. They may be worth more than you can imagine.

If you are a do-it-yourself kind of person, you can manage as much of the process of thinning out your possessions as you would like. There are excellent books written in response to the development of empty nesters. They range from downsizing your possessions to building a new downsized home.

Consider Your Home An Asset To Be Leveraged

Your home is usually one of your largest assets. Managing this asset can have a tremendous impact on self-determination and control as you age. The following are some items to consider. As families decrease in size and tastes in home layouts change, consider how to best leverage the sale of your home. The coming generation of families is generally smaller. The market for suburban single-family homes will shrink as the boomer generation sells off their primary family homes and supply increases. Do you want to be the home seller right in the middle of the huge home sell-off? As boomers age, the wave will ripple through the real estate market. Fewer and fewer buyers will be in the child-rearing phase and in the market for a traditional family-style home.

Your home may be in proximity to desirable urban areas or other strategic advantages like great schools. Consider carefully. Amenities you see as desirable—churches, libraries, playgrounds, etc.—may not appeal to your buyer. While the location of your home may be desirable, its design features may not. For example, a small master bathroom and eight-foot ceilings may weigh against you. You might consider selling early in the boomer age wave when values could be higher and inventory lower. When the boomers decide to sell as a market segment, the market will be flooded with three-bedroom, two-bath suburban homes. It might be wise to be on the front of the wave or get washed up with the gravel.

Downsizing to a smaller home earlier allows you to make your purchase decision closer to the current trends in real estate desirability. You would do much better to purchase a smaller home with an open floor plan, good light, and a more generous master bedroom and bathroom. It will be easier to sell in ten to fifteen years and appear far less "dated" than the 1970s brick ranch floor plan with a small kitchen and master bath. Given the number of single-person households due to divorce and later marriages, a residence with downsized features may be easier to sell should you move to a senior living community later.

Reverse mortgages can be a source of income in retirement. While I am not an expert on the process by any means, it bears consideration. If you have your plan in place, you can more easily determine the expected value of your home. Timing your mortgage in terms of peak value can impact your decision. It may be advisable to take the proceeds of a reverse mortgage, reinvest, and bank this asset, as certain classes of real estate (the bounteous 1970s brick ranch) may be in oversupply). Other investment options may be preferable to seeing your neighborhood "for sale" signs multiply as boomers transition. A bird in the hand...

Choosing the Right Downsized Home

Downsized residences, well chosen, may appeal to a broader market when you decide to move to senior living. Condos, cottages, and garden homes in well-placed locations appeal to the single-parent household, the young millennial generation, first-time home-buyers, and divorcees who have their children with them only part-time.

Values have changed. Younger buyers may place less value on square footage, yards, and swimming pools, preferring smaller residences with less upkeep. The millennial generation nurtures friendships and life experiences across electronic connections, not across the picket fence. Residence features are considered one component of a multi-dimensional lifestyle and not a predominant indicator of status or social class. With more people working from home and the desirability of access to urban conveniences, multi-family dwellings are now integrated into multiple-use developments. You often see "Work, Live, Play" promotional tag lines on mixed-use real estate developments where entertainment, retail, business, and shopping venues are built for convenience and community.

If you are no longer physically able to drive but cognitively intact, would you appreciate the walkability factor in a more urban area? If you are concerned about cognitive ability, understand that changing life patterns—shopping at a new grocery store, taking a left to church instead of a right, parking in the garage instead of on the street—can be easier to master while you are more physically and cognitively able to process the changes. I have seen ninety-two-year-olds, with significant cognitive impairment, live successfully in their family home of origin and struggle greatly with new environments. The appliance controls, the way the door swings, the amount of light coming into the window in the morning—these environmental factors have tailored your lifestyle and created familiar mental processes. Moving to a modern, unfamiliar floor plan with electronic thermostat controls and a host of other unfamiliar patterns can be difficult to master during the process of cognitive decline.

Choosing the Right Location

Consider your proximity to senior living, medical services, pharmacies, and wellness services as you age. Recent decades have seen migration toward urban areas. Small towns across America have seen main streets abandoned. Rural areas are challenged to maintain adequate health care providers, good public schools, hospitals, and employers. If this trend continues, access to aging services will be more difficult for people in rural areas.

All across the country, primary care physicians and independently owned physician practices have been consolidated into larger health care systems. With profitability considerations, lower-profit clinics and medical service locations are closed. Physician practices cannot survive on Medicare reimbursements combined with the longer service times needed for older patients. Fewer and fewer doctors are choosing geriatrics as a specialty. Primary care doctors are disappearing as medical students choose to specialize. Should you decide to move to senior living, does your current location provide access to a full range of quality senior living choices?

Recreation/Entertainment/Intellectual Stimulation

While having a cabin on the lake in a rural area may be great for your sixth decade, the beauty and isolation could become less desirable as you age. In my work in senior living, I have found that two components of life can almost universally be enjoyed by people of all ages: food and entertainment. While some of us do experience challenges with eating and mobility as we age, most people enjoy familiar music, entertainment, and food as other abilities for enjoyment may decrease. Consider your proximity to entertainment venues, restaurants you may enjoy, theaters, and shopping. If you plan to take classes in retirement, will you take online classes, join a CCRC (continuing care retirement community) with a lifelong learning program, or choose to live near a university?

Base Your Expectations on Your Own Reality

As we have discussed, retirement can be rewarding. It can also be a time of fear, apprehension, and dread if not handled with a positive, proactive attitude. It has been said that we do not fear death so much as we fear what happens to us before we die. Will we be disabled? Living with pain or illness? Will we have to give up our independence? Some seniors base their expectations of retirement on the experiences of their parents or grandparents. This is one of the most important pitfalls to avoid. Stereotypes of frail seventy-years-olds or male family members who expire in their early sixties can give us reason to relinquish planning or living our retirement years fully. We can have expectations that our families will cluster around us for barbeques, concerts, and holiday meals. Chances are, your retirement will only slightly impact the life patterns of your adult children as long as you remain independent. It is not uncommon to see seniors who have been sitting around waiting for twenty years only to find that they are healthy and have the potential for a vibrant lifestyle well into their nineties. It breaks my heart to see people with so much life to live passively waiting for something to happen.

Add Things to Your Life as Some Things Disappear!

As our peers age, we find that life can be filled with hospital visits, funerals, and loss through relocation. We have to be realistic about the challenges as well as the opportunities. Although we are dividing our subject matter into topics most relevant to children and topics most relevant to parents, hopefully you will read the entire book with an increased understanding of both perspectives.

Until you have experienced it, you cannot know the grief one experiences from the loss of friends due to death or relocation. Dynamics change drastically when couples who have been friends for decades lose a partner. The surviving partners may feel isolated. They may perceive that they no longer fit in because they are no longer part of a couple. Intact couples may struggle to reach out during the grief because of fear for their own situation. Patterns develop in long-term friendships that can be uprooted when one couple loses a partner. Think of all the things we may do in pairs—bridge, golf, and tennis. The absence of a partner changes these dynamics tremendously. There is no handbook for life transitions such as these. Remember that our current senior generation is accustomed to lifelong commitments, whether friendship, marriage, or partnership. Many people never imagine themselves apart from their spouses. Their identity is shattered, and they have few tools to reach out and form new social and support circles.

What to do? Focus your life plan on continually adding dimensions to your life as others diminish or disappear. Integrate into your life plan the continual pursuit of friendships and renewed or altered relationships. Pursue your personal interests, and you will be exposed to increasing numbers of persons such as yourself who are building a new life. The beauty of such a large component of seniors in our population is that you are everywhere! There are people just like you looking for new life experiences.

There is no need to be isolated due to a life transition. Never before have there been so many opportunities for older people to reach out and touch each other. There are fitness programs that cater to seniors. Investment clubs. Ballroom dancing organizations. Motorcycle clubs. Retired executives. Lifelong learning programs. Travel clubs. Blogs on the Internet that deal with a variety of retirement topics. Consumer groups such as AARP. Volunteer organizations. Church or synagogue groups. Senior Centers. Senior drop-in coffee shops with recreational programming. The choices are endless.

Grief and loss are inevitably going to be part of aging. A focused pursuit of new friendships is a strategy that will serve you well. You don't want to be the one waving as your neighbors leave their house for the last time and head off on a cross-country RV trip that lasts two years. You also don't want to have a closet of black suits and be the perpetual Rock of

Gibraltar at every memorial service in town. I am not being trite or insensitive, but you have to purposefully fill your life with positive pursuits to counterbalance the loss you may experience.

Plan for the Loss of Your Partner

If you are currently married or in a long-term relationship, you need to have a plan for the scenario when one partner's death precedes the other. Where will you live? How will your life patterns change? What will you do if you are the one left behind?

While you may jest about moving to a mother- or father-in-law suite in your son's backyard, think about the lifestyle this will provide. Will you be isolated in a new city and have to make an entirely new circle of friends? Is living in someone's home or backyard a situation that fits with your needs for privacy? While this approach has been popular in discussion, in reality, it can be a holding pattern—a life arrangement that you may not need now or ever. While your friends may not still live on your cul-de-sac, list the ones who are still in town. Are they in retirement communities? A condo downtown? If your social network is intact, relocation to be near family can separate you from your friends.

Moving to a backyard might make sense if your family is committed to providing end-of-life care for you and if your approach to family intimacy is such that neither of you would have it any other way. Moving in with family usually makes sense when a health condition renders this living arrangement a need rather than a desire. It can also make sense if Grandma loves experiencing life with extended family or would otherwise be living in an empty nest.

The idea is riddled with downside potential, however. Adult children may have to build or alter a home in order to accommodate mobility needs of the older person. Research into the appropriate construction, cost, and privacy concerns with multiple generations inhabiting a residential lot can be an intense exercise for space that may only be needed for a few years. Again, consider the opportunity cost. If you decide to relocate near family, there may be a lovely rental retirement community with a pool, fitness center, transportation, and, most of all, new friends to be made. As always, keep longevity in mind. Can you imagine yourself living in someone's backyard or guestroom for twenty years if that becomes the reality?

Self-Determination

While denial may delay some fear and apprehension about aging, it is always there. Hanging right over your head. I have been amazed in my career to see seniors explore continuing care retirement communities where care is a critical component of the product. They want to see the pool, the fitness center, the bar, the auditorium—anything related to the independent living component of the facility. When offered a tour of care levels such as memory care, assisted living, or nursing care, the answer is usually a flat and definitive "no!" No one wants to imagine being dependent on another. Our culture has defined independence as part of humanity. We are an individualistic society, and the need to depend on someone else is not what any of us imagine for our last months or years. Ignoring this possibility, however, is a serious pitfall.

The most important component of self-determination is education. How can you choose what is best for you unless you know what is available? Do you walk into a retail store, tell them your size, and let someone else choose what you will buy? While you may not need a new suit or dress, chances are that at some point you will need some form of senior living. Is the denial and fear really worth the consequence? Would you allow someone else to choose something that may be your home during a challenging period of life? I beg you not to let life happen to you. Transitioning to senior living can be an intense life event. It is of such a magnitude that few residents move out of a senior living arrangement once they move in, even if they are not happy with the place. You may no longer drive. Family can get busy. Your ability to change a choice that has been made for you is drastically decreased.

Transitioning to senior living can also be the best lifestyle decision one can make. Satisfaction rates with continuing care retirement communities exceed 90 percent when residents are surveyed after move-in. Remember, these are residents who took the task in hand, researched their options, and determined their future, fully in control of their destinies. I have no statistics to offer, but my experience tells me that satisfaction scores for residents who experienced a health crisis and who had a family member choose for them are far less stellar.

You may decide that you will not move to senior living unless it is need-driven. Many people do make this choice. Just know what you want and where you want to be when the need arises. During a health crisis, caregivers are dealing with Medicare, supplemental insurance, medications, therapy, and rehabilitation choices, not to mention their own life challenges, finances, and a host of other issues that have to be addressed. Do you really want someone else who is possibly not consumer savvy about senior living to make a choice for you in three to five days? If you ponder nothing else in this book, seriously consider my plea. To be dependent on others for care in a vulnerable situation with no power to change it could well be the worst consequence of procrastination you ever experience.

The good news is that senior living is not always in line with the stereotypes we imagine and fear. The industry has changed drastically in the last four decades. The choices are diverse and vary tremendously in quality, design, and service options. To assume that senior living is a bad choice and therefore avoid your research increases the possibility that you may end up living in the kind of retirement environment you fear most. Chances are, your loved ones may share your stereotypes, and should you have a crisis, you want to be in control.

As a parent, realize that it is your responsibility to determine your life plan. Procrastination and denial may create a crisis for you and for the one who has agreed to assist you with care. In fairness, if you don't determine what you want and plan for it, you must be grateful for what you get.

As with many stages of life, either you can make decisions or someone will make the decision for you. Worse yet, no one will make a decision, and denial and apathy can quickly erode the retirement foundation you have worked to create for so many years.

We hear euphemisms such as "The writing was on the wall," "It was right under your nose all along," "If it had been a snake, it would have bit you," and so on. We can hardly say we didn't know everyone was getting older. From consumer organizations that number in the millions, seeking to provide guidance on aging, to fledgling industries seeking to serve the coming age wave, the burgeoning population of seniors is upon us, with the boomers not far behind. Suffice it to say, the aging demographic is a powerful economic force that has not yet grown into its own power.

Engage the Help of Professionals

There is no substitute for the experience of professionals who deal with aging issues on a daily basis. Attorneys are an excellent resource for power of attorney, living wills and legal issues related to the management of your assets. Don't sign documents that you do not understand. Ask your attorney to review these items and explain the terms and consequences.

Social workers and geriatric care managers can help you explore options and determine the best fit for your needs.

They can also help you to assess personal struggles such as depression, grief and life engagement. Change is difficult and a compassionate ear can do much to assure you that challenges you face are shared by others around you. Telling your story to an objective resource lends new perspectives. We can become discouraged when we feel there are no alternatives that meet our need.

Financial advisors can help you to estimate your uses for assets during retirement years and plan accordingly. Look for advisors who hold professional certifications and are willing to provide counsel focused on your particular life situation rather than commission-based professionals who may have a vested interest in one scenario over another.

A great doctor is essential as a gatekeeper should you incur medical challenges. Don't be afraid to ask for referrals to specialists that deal with your particular issue. Your family doctor may enlist the help of geriatric psychiatrist or neurologist to provide expertise on cognitive issues. Having a good understanding of your condition is always preferable to the anxiety of not having all the information you need to make decisions. There is no shame in asking questions and consulting expert advice when you need it.

IV

Trends in Senior Housing Choices

From 1997 to 1999, we saw three years of increased senior housing construction to a point that the industry was overbuilt and struggled to keep adequate occupancy levels. With declining levels from the peak in 1999, we saw three decreasing years of construction, which eventually bottomed out in 2002. From 2002 to 2008, housing increased in gradual increments until the financial crash hit in 2008. From 2008 until the writing of this book in 2013, we have seen drastically low levels of new construction. The scarcity of capital and struggling occupancy rates have brought the market to a standstill. As it stands, the industry may never catch up to the eventual demand.

With all the hype about the coming wave of senior consumers, senior housing has a relatively low percentage of qualified elders who choose this option. Although larger numbers of people are age appropriate and financially capable of purchasing senior housing, a relatively small percentage of this qualified market chooses the product. With care needs increasing as we age, products such as assisted living and nursing care will see a higher market penetration because purchase of the product is need-driven.

Independent living, which is generally not need-driven, has seen intense challenges in the post-2008 economy. Fewer and fewer seniors are choosing to spend their assets, instead choosing to gather the wagons and wait until they need care. This "circle the wagons and wait" strategy has also impacted the assisted living and nursing care market, with families waiting longer and longer to make the move. With this pattern, you find shorter lengths of stay and much higher need levels among assisted and nursing care residents. This, of course, is a generalization to the broader market. You may find very independent residents in these care communities, depending on the philosophy or admission requirements of a particular community.

What does this mean to your family? While the construction boom from 1997 to 1999 was a bit hasty, we have now seen years of small increases in construction of senior housing. While capital markets are easing and we are starting to see increases in financing, we cannot ignore the fact that seniors are aging faster than the market can meet future demand. We will see new products developed that are designed to provide senior services without the brick-and-mortar component to fill the gaps. It can take eighteen months to build an average assisted living community and three years or longer to build more sophisticated campus-style products like a CCRC. Products designed to serve seniors where they live will increase. Whether seniors live in their family homes of origin, condos, or apartments, more services will come into play that do not include residence as a component of the product. The supply of quality, desirable senior residences may experience higher demand and thus put pressure on the consumer to commit early or expect the consequences of "no room at the inn" once a situation becomes need-driven. With nursing home construction at a virtual standstill, we can expect that the demand will outpace supply.

With the expansion of technologies such as medication and health monitoring services, emergency call systems for private homes, and in-person communication such as video monitoring, these services may start to fill the void. It will be interesting to see how preferences evolve as seniors face the possibility that residential care is not available. While not widely understood today, the impact of social interaction, lifestyle programming, and communal living seems to promote living stronger and longer. We discuss the value of social interaction later in the book under Reason #4: "I'll Cross That Bridge When I Get to It."

Where Are We Now?

Companies seek to serve the coming aging generation. Boomers seek to become literate about the subject of aging. Industries franchise themselves and develop corporate marketing strategies to reach the "mature market." And yet, sadly, many obvious truths "from the horse's mouth" go unheard and unheeded. My Top 10 Reasons (which are discussed beginning in the next chapter) are designed to further the dialogue between consumer and provider. Whether you see this book in an airport bookstore on the way to your next business destination or you receive it from a friend as a gift, my hope is that it makes life a bit easier, makes you feel more empowered, and gives you the words to discuss one of the hardest things we all face in today's society: getting older.

Like any life transition, growing older isn't always easy. It isn't always hard, either. So don't start pitying the "old people." In general, we have a pretty good life. We've learned a few things. Seen a few things. Been a few places, and yes, maybe we have a little money in the bank. Not always, but generally more than our parents had when they were our age, if they made it that far. We are living longer and better than prior generations. More challenged intellectually and physically. More engaged. And with far more choices for that third semester of years that so many of our parents did not get to enjoy.

With more years come more options, possibly more needs, and more consumption. With longer life sometimes comes frailty, and thus the need for living options not seen in prior generations.

That brings us to our topic at hand: With so many senior consumers needing some level of care, why do so few seniors "want" to go there? With "there" being "the home," "the senior living community," "the old folks home," assisted living, nursing care, or the CCRC.

For some of you industry professionals, these terms may get your bristle up. I am not big on the "F" word—that being facility—or "the home" or a lot of other terms you hear every day, but this book is for everyday people facing real challenges who often don't have an awareness of our politically correct language. You can insert community, or neighborhood, or whatever term makes you feel good, but we are here to have a real conversation with no stopping along the way for semantics or linguistic debate. So with Mom and Dad getting older and the need for altered living options becoming a reality, why do so many people not want to go "there"?

V
Cheeseburgers for Seniors

"Cheeseburgers for Seniors" is my catchphrase to describe the differences in the consumer preferences of the coming wave of seniors. The concept of the unique generation covers more than just longevity and intergenerational relationships. Seniors today are the first generation to experience life on demand. Because we are accustomed to microwave ovens, dishwashers, riding lawn mowers, and more, we generally want to do everything we do more efficiently and with more variety. If someone who came of age in the early 1900s were to hear a description of a microwave, that person would certainly not expect the unique generation's demand that these microwaves come in multiple brands, colors, sizes, and power levels if they can heat food in five minutes or less. One would expect that we would be thrilled for the convenience alone. Not so. We want it all, and to a surprising extent, we have been able to have it all.

The post-World War II generation has been willing to innovate, sacrifice, work tenaciously, and orchestrate one of the greatest generations known to man. Never before has one generation so thoroughly improved the quality of life of the Earth's inhabitants. It is not surprising that what we are willing to accept in senior living will have a monumental impact on the industry.

This brings us to our first reason that your parents don't want to move to senior living. It is a clear indicator that there is some disconnect between what seniors expect and some of the choices in the marketplace today. We expect food instantly, whether microwaved or fast food, upscale or sandwich. We are accustomed to having what we want and are willing to purchase it at the drop of a hat. Is it any wonder that one choice of cheeseburger at a retirement community for the rest of our lives doesn't quite cut it?

Reason #1: The Food Is Not Good!

As a consumer, I know I am going to be eating here most of the time for the rest of my life. So if I love cheeseburgers and have eaten five a month for the last twenty years, why would I want to move into a senior residence where the cheeseburgers are awful? This question has many dimensions that a son or daughter may never have considered. Why is a cheeseburger important?

Choice

While cheeseburgers may not be good for me, a cheeseburger of my choice and quality represents independence and self-determination. Our generation has lived life with the choice of cheeseburgers on demand. Good ones. Greasy ones. Double-decker ones. Boxed ones. Wrapped ones. And how many sauces, condiments, and sides have I been able to choose, almost 24/7 for the entirety of my adult life? Certainly, no generation before us has had the luxury of so many cheeseburger choices at the drop of a hat! As one who loves a good cheeseburger, I am grateful for living in America during a time of such abundance of choices. So no matter how good a cheeseburger may be, I don't want to have the choice of only one for the rest of my life!

Interesting how obvious this reason for resisting the move to senior living is, and yet ideas like this are often ignored. Having been a leader in the senior living industry for over twenty years, I have learned that there is a given outcome if you sit down to talk to twenty people living in a senior living community. At least fifteen will mention food. Ten of those will complain about it. Three will absolutely hate the food and have an opinion beyond what most of us want to hear. Residents of retirement communities talk to each other, their friends, and family constantly about food.

Even as a professional who loves, cares about, and has a passion for older people, I don't care to hear about how much salt was in yesterday's breakfast ever again. The reality is, as an industry, we are never going to be able to make gravy exactly like Aunt Emma or a cheeseburger like you grilled once in 1981 at the Fourth of July family barbeque. It just isn't possible to please everyone all the time. While we have things to learn, we can also process what Abe Lincoln said over a hundred years ago: you cannot please all of the people all of the time. A modern adaptation of a related quote—but you get my drift.

With that being said, in fairness to those tireless professionals who lovingly make the cheeseburgers, let's be real about cheeseburgers. Given that this may be the main event cheeseburger for the next years of life, can we really not make a great cheeseburger? I have heard every justification in the book for just plain old "bad food" in retirement communities. Taste buds age and become desensitized. Perception of temperature becomes dulled as we age. Heart-healthy options just aren't as tasty as you might otherwise get. Let's be real, folks. If you are in the hospitality business and this product is, in essence, the last cheeseburger your customer is going to get, you should be able to deliver a good cheeseburger.

While this may seem to be a contrived and convoluted dialogue, it isn't. As an industry, we have grown complacent in some areas with a captive audience of often need-driven consumers. For our customers, who need the care, security, and hospitality we provide, we often ignore one of the most important elements needed in order for a living situation to become "home." We ignore the consumer feedback when the consumers are right in front of us. Is it any wonder Mom doesn't want to move to senior living?

On-site focus groups (residents), complaining at a fever pitch about the poor quality of our product, are marginalized because we cannot deliver good food. Meanwhile, the sons and daughters of our customers struggle with parents who need care but repeatedly hear, "please don't put me in one of those places." How sad that later choices in life have become synonymous with losing control. Having to be "put" somewhere against our will because the choices are so unpalatable, we, as consumers, turn away and force someone else to make the decision for us by our avoidance, denial, or downright refusal to purchase what we need.

As a country of aging consumers, we need to elevate the dialogue about the role hospitality and quality of service plays in being served. As a theme of this book, we will continue to speak about choice. *Choice* in dining quality and options. *Choice* in care needs being met in ways that are valuable to us. *Self-determination* in whether to receive or pay for services we choose or don't choose.

Just as we as a country have to come to expect homogeneous, lifeless, grainy tomatoes as the norm in restaurants, we as consumers have come to expect less from senior living. Consumer education and involvement are key to exploring whether your perceptions are reality or fiction. Communicating your awareness and asking questions about factors that influence your decision will ultimately impact services provided. Senior consumers, by numbers alone, will have a drastic impact on the trends of the industry.

Consider a related consumer-driven food scenario: if we as a nation are going to continue to accept that tomatoes should be served on a salad, should we not demand real tomatoes? Or as an alternative, should we revolt and consistently refuse to buy tomatoes? We may insist that restaurants "hold the tomatoes" unless they are fresh, natural, flavorful, and not genetically engineered to be a consistent size, shape, and poor substitute for the tomatoes we used to know. What would happen if we refused all tomatoes until the quality we are offered improved? Tomatoes would change. Trust me. The farming industry is organized enough. If they can engineer a tomato to minute size variances so that tomatoes will fit in a shipping box in almost exact numbers every time and not spoil for countless days, they could find a way to fix the tomatoes.

Fortunately, great food in senior living is far more prevalent than are great tomatoes! With senior-living advertising budgets predominantly focused on getting you to come and take a tour, it is difficult to communicate good food through an ad. It is, however, very common for communities to offer you the opportunity to come and have a meal with them.

Consumers, both parents and adult children, are generally not experts in shopping for senior living until the need arises. This is too late to learn about the product. Unlike tomatoes, senior living is something we have never tasted before we start to visit and consider our options. And when Mom leaves, often because of death, we are too heartbroken and grief-stricken to rise up under our banner of experience and tell people what to expect. We are just too tired and too emotionally spent.

Finding a Community with Good Food

So if we are considering buying senior living and we know the number one consideration is food, how do we shop? Of primary importance is to shop early. Shop *before* we need the product. As a family, discuss the possibilities and explore the options. There are great communities that serve great food, from delicious regional cuisine in "down home" communities to formal, elegant, full-course dining experiences in communities from Florida to California. If you encounter a larger national provider that does not design menus to fit local tastes, explore a smaller, regional company or nonprofit in your region that *does* have fare designed close to home.

You will find senior living communities that outsource hospitality services such as dining to companies that specialize in food production. This could be a consideration in your choice. While you might hope that you could determine quality based on a food services management contract provided by Company A, Company B, or internal management, you cannot. Ultimately, the cost of raw food and staffing levels is determined by the community, not the outsourced vendor. As with any organization, leadership and staff continuity at the local level is a strong driver of excellent product delivery. *Customization* to regional or cultural taste preferences is important. *Variety within the menu cycles* is certainly among the top considerations.

Menu cycles can range from two weeks to six weeks, with some organizations having multiple menu cycles. If multiple menu cycles are employed, it allows for the use of seasonal ingredients that are available fresh during certain times of the year. Longer menu cycles with multiple menu cycles available for production, definitely detract from the monotony of eating in the same restaurant every day. For example, you might have a six-week menu cycle designed for fall and winter. This six-week cycle might repeat twice and then be replaced with a menu cycle including the fresh fruits and vegetables of the spring and summer. As a prospective resident, your perception of the taste, quality, and variety is the ultimate determining factor.

If you determine that food is one of your top ten reasons for avoiding senior living, here are some strategies aimed at investigating food-related factors that are most important to you.

Don't wait until your demand for the product (senior living) exceeds your time and capacity to shop the options in your area. Connect with the staff and go have a cheeseburger! Have a meal. Often, senior living communities will provide complimentary meals for prospective families. One meal is probably not enough. Your parent or loved one may absolutely refuse to visit with you. Go anyway. Chances are that if your loved one is avoiding the decision, this behavior may continue well beyond his or her ability to make an independent choice. Health or safety issues may necessitate that you make or participate in the choice for your parent(s). Since health or safety crises can be stressful on the family dynamic, you will be happy you got to know the choices before you suddenly needed the product.

Make friends with a resident. The best consumer review is one from a trusted source. Learn about senior living communities where your friends, former colleagues, or fraternal groups live. Offer to pay the guest meal charge to dine with your friend. This gives him or her a lovely dining experience to enjoy and allows you to become a more informed consumer. Trust me. Your friends will enjoy you coming to be with them. They will tell you their honest opinion of how they like the place. If nothing else, age often gives us honesty and forthrightness not seen in our younger years.

Drop in. For breakfast. For dinner. For lunch. In the afternoon after the big holiday buffet. What happens on holidays when a residence generally experiences lower staffing levels and is rebounding from a large dining offering? Are managers on duty? Does it seem like an inconvenience to accommodate an additional guest? When hospitality and warmth is a primary concern, what reaction would you expect when a guest drops in? Observe the response. Are staff members worried about not having enough food? This may indicate a slim production margin for food. The lack of ability to accommodate one or two more guests could indicate that food costs are held low and that variety may be monotonous or nonexistent to control food costs.

Order from the alternative menu. Most quality senior-living communities offer alternative menus at every meal. This often includes a sandwich, or soup and salad to provide variety and choice. Again, how reasonable these offerings are is key. Don't expect to order a filet mignon to temperature. It is reasonable to expect some type of upscale alternative order. It is just not the norm in today's world. If you are fortunate enough to encounter an enlightened menu system with an offering such as this, gladly pay the additional charge for the upgrade and rest comfortably knowing that, for some appreciative residents, this option is a cherished blessing when the routine calls for a special treat. We cannot expect to pay for premium products as a component of an otherwise middle market offering at a basic rate to the resident.

Have a meal in an area where care is provided. This may need to be prearranged in a conversation with sales staff in the community. Just let them know that you are interested in the assisted living, nursing, or memory care areas, and at some point in the future, you may drop in to have a meal with the residents. Document the conversation and follow through. If your drop-in seems unwelcome or an inconvenience, consider carefully before you write the deposit check. However, be aware that drop-ins are not common. Most caregivers prize compassion, and, especially in the case of nurses, perfection. Having three sisters who are nurses in addition to decades of experience with nurses as colleagues, I have found that it is rare to find care staff who don't want to help you. Caregivers may be stressed. They may be poorly trained. They may have another resident who just had a fall on their minds, but rarely do you find someone in this profession who is uncaring.

There is a difference between staff being somewhat taken aback by a new visitor and acting put upon by the added visitor, making that person feel unwelcome. Unfortunately, visitors at mealtimes are not a common occurrence. Most senior living communities create family nights or themed parties where visitors are welcomed and encouraged to spend time with their families in a festive mode. Staff may be accustomed to these venues and feel unprepared to welcome a guest in other circumstances. After some adjustment from the staff and a positive, friendly attitude from you, the experience should go well. If anything, staff in senior living are accustomed to new situations. If you have ever tried to give someone with cognitive impairment and a fear of water a bath, you have some idea of what I mean.

Some communities offer multiple levels of care, starting with independent living and moving through a range of options to the highest level of care provided in a nursing home, assisted living, or other regulated area. Independent living generally provides housekeeping services, home maintenance, dining and retail options, and convenience services such as spa, salon, transportation, and travel.

When residents need assistance with activities of daily living (ADLs), most states require that they engage a higher level of care, either through moving to a regulated area of the building or campus or by bringing services into their independent living residence. Suffice it to say, independent living residents are often the most vocal and demanding consumers. You will generally find more attention paid to dining quality, options, and venues for independent living residents, and less importance placed on these components as residents' care needs increase. Given this information, it is very indicative to have a meal where care is provided such as assisted living or nursing care.

Confirm which dining venues are available to your care situation. Independent living dining venues may have a lovely Sunday "jazz brunch." Are residents in care levels and their families welcome in this dining venue? Is there a charge system in place, resident billing, or may visitors pay with a credit card?

Ask questions about the amount budgeted for food. Moving to a senior living community is a life choice on the magnitude of marriage, divorce, a career change, the birth of a child, or the death of a family member. Treat it as such. You deserve to have your questions answered to the extent and detail that make you comfortable with the decision.

Most senior living communities track the expense of caring for residents in minute detail. There is an industry term—per resident per day (PRPD)—that details expenditures on everything from cleaning supplies to raw food costs. While cleaning supplies may not be your utmost concern, you probably do want to know what the community is spending on the food you or your mom will be eating. As of the writing of this book, the lowest raw food cost per resident per day I have seen is three dollars per day. A low raw food cost is not a good indicator. If you can imagine yourself purchasing the raw ingredients to prepare three full meals for three dollars per day, you can also imagine what those meals might contain. Not too much of any great quality. Raw products for breakfast food are often less expensive to purchase, and you may see these provided at other mealtimes for communities only spending three dollars per day on meals. You may also see processed meat products that are questionable in content, such as hotdogs, breaded meat patties, and high sodium sandwich meats. Look for soups that recur daily on the menu that use high-sodium, packaged, powdered soup base.

Some communities provide soup and sandwiches as their evening meals, and this is not necessarily an indication of a low raw food cost. Residents generally do prefer having their larger meals at the noon hour. For people whose physical activity has decreased, a light meal in the evening is often enough. Skipping meals is not a good idea, and it is best to have something in the evening that is light and will be desired. When residents take multiple medications, the digestive tract needs food to facilitate the body's processing the medications taken in the evening and before bed.

You would expect a minimum of seven dollars per resident per day in raw food costs in assisted living or nursing care. With creative and committed dieticians and kitchen staffs, one could imagine a good product being delivered. You must also remember that senior living communities purchase in volume and get discounts not available to non-institutional consumers. This discount can impact what a community needs to spend to deliver a quality product. Consider logic and reason when discussing the issue.

In independent living areas, the dollar amounts may be harder to track, given that often only one meal is delivered to residents. Kosher communities will see much higher amounts spent on food. Purchasing kosher meats and dairy products can be quite expensive. If you are exploring a kosher community, you might expect to see a 35-percent increase in daily raw food costs. While this measure can give you some indication of the quality of the food provided, nothing replaces tasting the finished product to determine quality.

As we will discuss later in the book, different living options provide different levels of care, and associated costs can fluctuate among types of care. As we age, we generally do eat smaller portions. With some seniors who are less active, their bodies require fewer calories to accomplish their daily physical activity. Digestive systems can also become sluggish. With movement and activity, your body operates in the way it was designed to operate. With less activity, systems can slow down.

If you have had much experience with the very elderly, sedentary senior, you know that laxatives can become a focus of life. While this may be a topic only less desirable to discuss than bad food, it becomes important. Constipation definitely has an effect on your energy level and mood. Medications or combinations of them can often decrease appetite or cause constipation. Suffice it to say that portions consumed by residents in assisted living or nursing care will be less than those in an independent setting, and thus the corresponding raw food costs will be lower.

Ask questions about nutrition and the variety of foods served. Regulatory agencies generally stipulate how many ounces of protein, starch, and vegetables should be provided for residents, and a staff dietician ensures nutritional compliance. In my experience, this amount is generally adequate or even beyond what elder seniors want to consume. I have never experienced a senior living community that was not thrilled to have a resident request second helpings or even thirds if initial servings are not enough. Sometimes, meal choices are not appetizing due to personal or regional tastes or the structure of menu choices can be repetitive and boring. When dining becomes a highlight in your day, you quickly learn the pattern. It can also be the case that the menu is so mundane or the food quality so poor that residents just don't care to eat hamburger steak yet again for the fourth time in a month. It is good to have menu cycles that change periodically.

You can expect that assisted living and nursing care menus will contain what we in the industry call "comfort food." In this generation, these items are often foods that present-day seniors traditionally ate growing up, are easy to digest, and give one a sense of home. Examples might be meatloaf and mashed potatoes, beef stroganoff, hamburger steak with gravy, or liver and onions. These offerings should vary regionally based on what residents from that area of the country would enjoy. You will see far more meat and potatoes in the Midwest, or gravy, gumbos, and fried chicken in the Deep South. You will find matzo ball soup in West Palm Beach catering to the vast number of New York and New Jersey residents who have migrated to Florida in their active adult years. Clam chowder and lobster rolls are naturally common in New England. Vegan offerings will be more prominent in California menus. Communities that cater to Asian residents might serve four or five kinds of rice. Many comfort foods have a gravy or liquid component that can help provide a more tender, digestible protein for senior consumption. Meats steamed or cooked in gravy tend to be more moist and tender than dry pieces of meat.

Although I cannot prove that residents prefer comfort food at later stages in life, I have seen the process in action through my twenty years of experience. As we grow older, we want to experience those feelings of home and family connection. Food is a great platform for creating this sense of nurturing. With time to consider earlier stages of life, we come to associate many of those memories with a pleasant food experience. The smell of bacon frying in the pan. Chicken boiling on the stove with celery, onions, and garlic in preparation for soup on a cold winter day. The smell of matzo brie cooking in the oven on Friday morning. Food can be a contributing factor in making one feel home and welcome.

For residents who have cognitive impairment, food smells can stimulate the appetite and signal that it is time to have a meal. As memory declines, other senses help residents to evaluate the world around them. We know that sensory stimulation outside ourselves activates a process of recognition through neural pathways in the brain. Often these maps created through neural pathways can be paired with another sensory experience. Smells with food. Touch with caring or nurturing. Smiles when all is well. It is a vast and only slightly researched method of communication for those with cognitive impairments.

Life Example - *It can be quite miraculous when you stumble upon one of these sensory triggers. I saw one of these miracles unfold before my eyes. In one of the communities I managed, we had the joy of caring for a lovely lady who had loved to dance in her younger years. Let's call her Jane. With the progression of cognitive impairments and the side effects of medication, her walking gait had become shortened and belabored. Her steps were short in distance, and she shuffled, barely picking up her feet as she moved. This is sometimes called the Parkinson shuffle—a mobility issue that you see in people who have Parkinson's disease. It almost appears as if the hip joints are frozen and it is impossible for the person to extend his or her leg to move the full length of a footstep. Needless to say, Jane did not move fluidly, and it took great effort and time to navigate even short distances.*

One evening, we had a big band from the community perform for dancing and entertainment. Jane attended, and her brother came to join her. They had both been avid dancers in their younger years, and you could see the expression of joy on her face. No one had any expectation that with her impaired mobility she would be able to dance. It just didn't seem possible. Her brother asked her to dance not knowing how well she would be able to participate. Talk about a miracle! Her feet started to move to the music. Her legs moved in normal sequence and spacing, with the distance of her steps increasing. She was quickly gliding along the dance floor to an old Tommy Dorsey tune. She danced beautifully! Her learning of dance was paired with the musical sensory stimulation, and thus her movements were learned through different neural pathways. She was able to dance using this learned memory processed in an area of the brain that had not been damaged through disease. There were many tears of joy and hope in the room that evening.

I use this story to illustrate that aging—and, certainly, senior living awareness—is a journey. There were no family members or staff who *could have predicted nor orchestrated this outcome of joy. The approach, however, of walking the talk by engaged severely memory-impaired residents in live music events is key. We cannot relegate memory-impaired residents to what we think or expect to be their capabilities. In resident-centered care, we discover, through relationship, our residents' abilities and capacities for joyous moments.*

Additional Questions to Ask about Dining Services

The questions below will help you determine if dining continues to be an enjoyable experience for residents or is merely a clinical exercise in nutrition.

- Do residents who need help still have lovely, palatable choices?

- Ask to see the menus for the last three months. Most communities keep them on file. Is the same menu repeating every week or every three weeks? Do they have seasonal menu cycles that take advantage of fresh fruits and vegetables when in season?

- Is wine available with meals here? Is a physician's order required to order alcoholic beverages? What about happy hour?

- Is the alternative menu as comprehensive as in other care areas?

- Are meals prepared on-site nearby, or are they transported from production kitchens in other areas of the building or campus?

- Are tables well appointed? Are tablecloths replaced and linens clean and well maintained? Visit between meals.

Are crumbs in the chairs? Are tables reset with a clean dining area between meals? Staff expected to provide both care services and hospitality services, such as waiting tables, often must leave the meal and provide personal care to residents afterward. If staffing is stretched or poorly managed, you might see dining areas still not cleaned midmorning or afternoon. Communities that use caregiving staff to assist with meals call this a "universal worker" model. This model is designed to simulate natural family patterns and strong awareness of the needs of the residents. It can also be a cost-saving measure with little training provided to the caregiver in dining etiquette and service expectations.

- Are residents who need assistance with dining treated in a dignified manner? Is staff providing assistance? Are they working with one or multiple residents? Is cross contamination an issue? Staff assisting multiple residents must prevent transfer of germs from one resident to another. Privacy? You never want to see medications doled out at meals or in any other public venue. Residents talk.

- Take a tour of the kitchen. Is the space adequate? Does equipment appear to be broken or poorly maintained? Are floors clean? Are trash cans away from areas where they could come in contact with food?

- How are low sodium and low sugar diets monitored? Are pictures of residents who have food allergies or restrictions posted *behind the scene* so that wait staff know which residents need special precautions taken with their food? These photographs combined with resident profiles should only be in view of staff in private employee areas. Is the area organized and clean?

- Are juices and beverages prepared fresh, or are they dispensed from a machine that mixes the ingredients? There has been a never-ending pursuit in senior living to come up with a product that resembles fresh, vibrant juices with a dispenser that is convenient and easy to clean. If you choose a community with dispensers, are the nozzle heads and levers that deliver the product clean and free of product buildup? You will be able to tell if these machines are clean and being maintained daily.

- Are linens changed after each meal? What measures are taken to prevent the transfer of germs from one meal to the next, or from one resident to another? Do the linens match, or does there seem to be a shortage? Problems here can indicate stringent cost controls, poorly coordinated or managed housekeeping staff, or a lack of focus on the hospitality component of senior living.

- Investigate starting pay rates for dining staff, nursing assistants, and nurses. The industry generally employs large numbers of low-wage staff, and low wages don't always mean poor care. Most staff have a high compassion level that draws them to the industry. If, however, the norm in your area for nursing assistants is nine dollars per hour and the community you are researching pays minimum wage, you might expect high turnover or staff who have other primary jobs and work at this location for secondary income. Senior living staffers tend to have compassion in abundance, and they often end up being the primary financial caregivers for their families. Staff members working two jobs are often stretched thin and have less to give when they get to their secondary jobs. Conversely, communities who employ part-time workers for second jobs during peak periods for four hours per shift can indicate progressive and enlightened management. Meal service and medication assistance generally cluster around the morning, noon and evening meals. Employing extra part-time staff for four hours surrounding these events can support quality and efficient care at reduced costs to you, the consumer.

- Ask about scheduling for staff. Do they work twelve-hour shifts? Eight hours? Flexible staffing, in which staff might work in four-hour increments? Twelve hours is a long day for work that involves high physical and emotional demands. Caregivers working from 6:00 a.m. to 6:00 p.m. are expected to provide daily care upon their arrival, often serving breakfast and lunch and providing medication assistance for the two medication passes aligned with breakfast and lunch. They can work four twelve-hour days in a row, which can be very stressful. Some providers employ this strategy to avoid open positions on the second shift—2:00 p.m. to 10:00 p.m., or 3:00 p.m. to 11:00 p.m. While this may seem to solve the problem of poor attendance, it can leave a well-staffed team burned out and overworked from multiple twelve-hour shifts. You cannot use any one factor as a determinant to judge a community rotten or excellent. My questions enable you to have a broader picture of the entire operation.

- You may indecd find nursing staffs who work twelve-hour shifts because they actually voted to move to this system. If so, this shows an extreme amount of responsiveness to employees by the company. There are twelve-hour shift scenarios where one works only a maximum of three days in a row. Some scenarios include combinations of twelve-, eight-, and four-hour shifts by part-timers. I have used four-hour shifts in the morning on both sides of breakfast and dinner to help with personal care, dining, and medication assistance. This provides for added staff members on the roster in case of absence. It also provides for a break between work periods. At one point, I had a husband and wife share one full-time job through this system, and it worked quite well for their family.

Memory Care Considerations

Are special systems in place to encourage pleasant dining? These might include the following:

- Contrasting service ware colors may help visually impaired residents distinguish table linens from utensils and food from serving plates.

- Are there plates that create a contrasting background so that food can be located and identified on the plate? White plates against a dark linen color allow residents to perceive the plate outline and food color against the white plate.

- Diners who wander should be provided with "finger food" or appetizer-style options if they cannot sit still.

- Many communities provide eat-on-the-go versions of the same meals provided to sit-down diners. These foods can often mirror their plate-served counterparts, such as chicken cordon bleu prepared as a finger food or an appetizer.

- Are residents eating the food they are provided?

- Are dining environments quiet and well lit, allowing residents to focus on eating? Sounds of clattering dishes, verbalizing from the kitchen, and doors opening and closing can distract those with limited cognition. Any situation that distracts or overstimulates a cognitively impaired resident is going to hinder a quality dining experience.

- Do staff members adjust their communication to give direct eye contact to residents? Do they speak *to* residents or *about* them? Do they use sentences of seven words or fewer so that communication can be processed and understood by residents with cognitive impairment?

It is often a natural response to ask questions about low sodium or no-added-salt diets. Communities promote healthy alternative menu choices. Meals in pureed or modified form are offered for those who have physical problems with swallowing. The bottom line from a happiness perspective is resident enjoyment. You cannot know how happy a hot dog might make you if you have not been to a ballpark for ten years. Yet you should also be aware that hot dogs served multiple times per week may indicate scrimping on food costs.

One of my passions is quality, enjoyable food. Don't put a rib eye on the menu and give me something that is of such poor quality and toughness that it is not enjoyable. All of us hate to feel duped or a victim of the old "bait and switch," whether we are thirty or eighty. It just doesn't create a level of trust and caring when this happens.

I'd rather have an A-plus, top-notch meatloaf that smells like heaven coming from the kitchen every Friday night than a rib eye on the menu that just leaves me feeling cheated and lied to. You think this sounds like good, pragmatic common sense, right? Wrong. As a senior-level executive, I was a participant in a meal provided by a senior living dining services management company. They were pitching senior-level executives for an opportunity to obtain the contract to provide food services. Two of their finest chefs had been flown in from across the country for the on-site presentation. One of the options provided was a rib eye salad. The beef was inedible. With my middle-aged physical capacity, I could neither chew nor taste the product that had been prepared. I had no delusions that any of my eighty-plus-year-old residents might enjoy it. Needless to say, they didn't get the contract. Nor did I finish the rib eye salad. Quality is measureable to the senses. Don't be fooled by the lovely website photos with models in chef hats. Invariably, you will see the famous and overused "Chef's Special Soup." This could mean that he or she made the soup with the "special" from yesterday that did not sell and was left over. Beware of sizzle without any steak. Sample the merchandise.

VI

Operations and Safety Considerations

Reason #2: It Smells Bad!

For many years, the telltale sign of a poorly managed, low-quality senior living home has been the smell of urine. While I hope this goes without saying, if you encounter the smells of bodily functions as a pervasive overlay of the environment, run, don't walk, out of there. While accidents do happen, encountering the smell of waste of any sort should not be a regular experience. Should you be on a tour of even the best community, you may pass an apartment door or a soiled linen area that could provide an unpleasant smell. If, however, the smell is pervasive, the home probably has a poor level of care and a systemic problem. Good senior living communities address hygiene needs promptly. Training programs teach staff to double-bag used, disposable undergarments and quickly take them to a designated area. They should be removed at the end of each shift.

"Stink" is a relative term. We all know it when we smell it. Stink can be antiseptic, chlorinated, pine-flavored, or even potpourri. Bad smells can be obvious, or they can be camouflaged. Take into consideration what your loved ones might perceive. An antiseptic smell may mean that they are comforted by a scent they relate to cleanliness. Pine cleaner smells give me a sense of a freshly cleaned house. I love to walk into a home that has recently been thoroughly cleaned with a pine cleaner. I have visited nursing homes providing the absolute highest intensity of care and compassion available that smell antiseptic. While I personally would not want to live there, I would have utmost confidence in picking up a chicken tender in the hallway and eating it even beyond the five-second rule!

Trust your gut. Trust what you experience. Look for evidence of "walking the talk." Any good senior living establishment should smell like a home—like delicious food, fresh-cut flowers, even the local sweaty kids' soccer team romping in from their latest game to visit, volunteer, and celebrate. You know what real life smells like. Senior living is real life, and it can be just as rich and dimensional as your mudroom on a Saturday morning. Don't let produced fragrances or expectations overcome your initial reaction to the feeling and sense of home you experience in a good, community-integrated senior living facility. It will smell like the activities of the original residence of the residents who live there on any given day at any given time, but it *should not* smell like urine or other filth or waste by any means.

Assess the Housekeeping

Common areas should be clean and inviting. I have always been passionate (my former staff might say obsessive) about keeping doors and entryways inviting. If you approach a smudged, dirty, glass-paned door that hasn't been cleaned in a week, how comfortable would you be with the staff taking care of your loved one? I use the same rule when approaching restaurants. If the food is as clean as the door, am I still OK to eat it? If not, I head back to the parking lot. Senior living is not just about care. It is about hospitality and a feeling of home.

A word of clarification: hospitality, cleanliness, and a sense of home are not about how recently the building was built.

New buildings may mean that an organization has held true to its mission and core values and is thus experiencing more demand. That's true. But not always. Running a senior living community is about making the best of what you have. I have seen multimillion-dollar buildings go poorly maintained and become worn and smelly after only a few years of operation. Conversely, I have seen antiseptic-smelling cinder-block buildings in rural areas provide the best genuine love and compassion on the market. It is also the case that employee retention may be better in a rural area. If there are few jobs, and senior living provides a career path of security and stability, you may well find some of the best nurses, cooks, and housekeepers in the business—many of whom have been with the company for five, ten, and even forty years! I have noticed this in many rural areas in the South as well as in the Midwest. While sparsely populated by East or West Coast standards, states like North and South Dakota, Kansas, and Colorado have excellent care choices. This brings me to our next topic—staffing.

Staffing Acquisition and Retention

Although upscale suburbs may be desirable for single-family dwellings, the cost of living and poor public transportation connections may make for challenging staff retention. Senior living facilities must have an accessible work force nearby. Consider this when choosing between one location or another. If Choice A has a predominance of family who live or work in an area that is more conducive to attracting good staff, and if Choice B is next door to the neighborhood of origin, Choice A may be the winner. You may also consider the kinship between the residents of Choice B in the neighborhood of origin. If friends have moved into this community, the existing relationships to current residents might outweigh the staffing considerations. Price can also come into play. The land value of a desired location can impact the monthly service fees.

It is not uncommon for nursing care organizations to experience turnover rates in excess of 100% per year. Understanding that continuity of care is crucial, turnover of this magnitude often indicates inconsistent care. As residents age, understanding of their preferences, personal care routines and corresponding medical conditions can best be accomplished by stable and well-trained staff. Many communities strive to maintain staff consistently assigned to the same residents on an on-going basis. Does the community use outside staffing to fill open positions and absences? These are usually nurses or nursing assistants who work for an agency and are provided to supplement permanent workers. While this is not always an indicator of problems, many communities do not allow agency usage due to inconsistency in care and costs.

With day shifts desired by most workers, second shift or overnight positions can turnover frequently. Senior living can be a highly stressful work environment due to the demands and frailty of residents. It is important that senior living organizations provide an affirming, nurturing and supportive environment to retain high quality staff.

Observe interactions between supervisors, managers and community leadership. Are line staff addressed on a first name basis and treated with dignity and respect? Are programs in place to recognize excellent performers? It is certainly appropriate to ask questions about staff tenure. Most organizations monitor this statistic yearly. Tenure of managers is also a relevant question. Unfortunately, leaders who have served three or more years in management positions are the exception rather than the norm. Make a special effort to meet the Executive Director or Administrator of the community you are considering. Evaluate their compassion and comfort level with your questions. Leadership determines the culture and mission of the organization.

Take Note of the Parking Facilities

As you drive into the parking lot, it should be clean and free of trash, with handicapped or accessible parking near the building. There may be times when you have groceries or supplies that have to be delivered to the apartment and you don't want to walk a mile to get them there. In an effort to be accessible to residents in their home neighborhoods or to the residents' adult children, senior living companies can choose locations that, due to land costs or topography, are not able to provide adequate turning space for residents or convenient loading and unloading. This may not be the make-or-break factor for deciding upon a community, but it is good to make a note of how much you are willing to overlook in parking.

Urban locations often do the best they can while trying to build a sufficient number of units to afford the convenience of the location. A large percentage of assisted living communities provide a covered area for loading and unloading. Independent living communities should provide accessible parking for their residents. An independent senior will be doing many of the same errands and activities he or she has done forever. Imagine how convenient the parking would be if you needed the assistance of a walker or wheelchair. Are there adequate spaces to load and unload the assistive devices? Is handicapped parking accessible? How is the distance to the apartment? Navigating stairs, elevators, uneven or poorly lit areas, or heavy doors can be difficult with an assistive device.

When Considering Senior Living Communities

- Ask about parking allocations. Are residents allowed to keep cars on premises?

- Are parking areas well planned, with generous turning space and sight lines free of shrubbery or obstructions?

Remember, these are the professionals. Planning for aging functionality and convenience should be inherent in design for senior living.

- Are parking areas accessible to the residence? Consider walking distance, lighting, and climate control for access when returning with groceries or packages.

- What are the policies for residents on driving and maintaining cars on property? This is a safety issue for you and your family as well. While your loved one may well be self-aware and conscientious in driving safety, what are the requirements and benchmarks for other residents who choose to drive? At what point does management step in to maintain a secure environment for all?

- Are residents required to provide proof of auto insurance and a valid driver's license if driving on campus?

Is it time to stop driving?

Cognitive function assessments such as the mini-mental inventory and guidance by your physician are valuable tools to evaluate safety issues. Cognitive function can be measured objectively. Pre-determined agreements developed with the advice of your medical provider can provide benchmarks when driving is no longer safe. Some vision impairments can be reversed by medical procedures such as removal of cataracts. There are now "virtual driving simulators" that can measure reaction time and capability in simulated scenarios. Senior health clubs such as Nifty after Fifty (www.niftyafterfifty.com) use theses simulators to help us gauge our ability to continue to drive. Occupational therapists can also provide guidance in this area.

While your mother or father is healthy and in control of his or her geographic whereabouts, listen to the markers that indicate that your parent should no longer drive. Be aware. Driving is not always about the actual act of driving. Driving is an indicator of *choice* and *self-determination*. You can often only access those multiple cheeseburger life-choices with wheels at your command. With your loved one, predetermine the markers that may indicate choices. AARP safe driving classes for seniors help to create awareness of personal capacity. Physicians can be a credible resource to assist in identifying danger in continuing to drive. Collaborate to create a scenario in which your loved one makes his or her choice according to a predetermined parameter. The worst scenario is for a loved one to be involved in accidents where either your loved one or someone else is injured. "Taking away the keys" means a blow to choice and self-determination in addition to possible feelings of guilt if someone is harmed.

Fire Safety

Add fire safety systems to your list of environmental considerations. Newer buildings may use sophisticated digital display panels to track and indicate where smoke, sprinkler heads, or fire sensors have triggered. Digital panels are often located near the front door so that all occupants of the building can view the alarm panel. Some communities locate these panels within maintenance areas. It is crucial that staff be thoroughly trained on the procedures to effectively use these systems and have access to the panels. Systems may provide a digital outline of building areas with blinking lights indicating the floor and area of the alarm. Systems with this level of sophistication generally have installed retractable fire walls that allow a certain area of the building to avoid evacuation and be protected from smoke. Residents may remain in their fire-wall-protected area of the building for four hours in some cases without evacuation.

State regulatory agencies generally require fire drills on all shifts at least twice per year with some states mandating quarterly fire drills on each work shift. Documentation of and attendance in these drills is kept for state regulatory visits, training documentation, and performance tracking.

Older buildings may only provide fire sprinkler systems and smoke detection with no monitoring of the area alarmed. Fire sprinkler systems are very effective. While a sprinkler system alone may not provide you the luxury of staying in your protected, fire-walled area while the affected area evacuates, it will save your life. You may end up wet with some damage to your property, but being wet and alive is always preferable to other options! This is a good example of why renter's insurance is a good idea when living in senior living communities.

Some buildings may be grandfathered and not required to provide sprinkler systems due to age and cost of retrofitting the building. Many group homes are also not required to provide sprinkler systems. However, they generally house smaller numbers of residents in single-story buildings with less distance to exits, and have higher ratios of care staff to residents. You can see how one caregiver could more easily evacuate six residents from a residential one-story building vs. one caregiver responsible for ten residents in a multiple-story building with stairwells.

Fire safety requirements vary from state to state, and multiple-level buildings tend to require more sophisticated fire-evacuation procedures. Always consider the sophistication of the system in conjunction with overnight and weekend staffing levels and the number of floors and size of the building. Fire safety oversight in senior living is generally regulated by both the state regulating agency for senior living and the Department of Fire Safety, either local or state.

Natural Disasters

Having led senior living organizations in both Louisiana and California, it is prudent to consider scenarios where emergency response measures are necessary. Whether hurricanes, earthquakes, tornadoes, floods or other natural disasters, you or the community you choose will have to provide support, and provide guidance and leadership in an emergency situation. Explore possible scenarios. Will family members be able to provide evacuation and housing should the community have to be evacuated? Whether mandated by local governmental authorities or just good judgment, there are scenarios where a senior living community must be evacuated.

When evacuation is not mandated, consider the implications of disasters on remaining housed in the community. Ask questions about power generating capacity. How are generators fueled? What time period is covered by emergency power resources? Are generators allocated to emergency call systems, climate control or production facilities for food? What supply of emergency food rations is held at the community?

While this may seem complex, states that are prone to natural disasters generally require senior living communities to provide regulatory agencies with their emergency plans. You can request a copy. Such plans often include housing in place strategies as well as evacuation destinations if necessary. Regulatory oversight dictates increasing emergency preparedness measures as the level of care or frailty increases. For example, a nursing home may be required to provide more comprehensive emergency power for medical equipment than is necessary for independent or assisted living. Remember that independent living is designed to house residents who are "independent" and expected to fully execute or participate to some extent in emergency preparedness. It is good to be clear on resident and family responsibilities related to the level of care provided by the community. While some residents desire to remain in independent living well past the level of services provided in independent living, this approach comes with inherent risks in a disaster scenario. While transportation, food service and provision of personal and medical care in a disaster may be provided for assisted living, memory care and nursing care residents, independent living residents are generally not covered for these services.

Personal Safety

Many senior living campuses have gated, secured access systems that require electronic access. Some have gatehouses that are staffed twenty four hours per day with lists of guests and vendors approved to access the community. Newer communities that are adopting concepts of the new, mixed use, urban planning may have retail or public access spaces such as cafes, health clubs or meeting areas open to the community with limited access to residential areas. There are pros and cons of both open and closed community approaches. While you may feel more secure in a controlled access community, younger residents may prefer a more integrated community model where they encounter a broader variety of personal interactions. Some communities have multi-generational programs for child care or after school tutoring or mentoring programs. Many communities now open their services to seniors who have not yet moved into residence at the community. This may also be the case if your community offers "virtual care" for seniors still living in their own homes. These community members may access medical, wellness or dining services on the campus while still living at home. We will cover virtual CCRC's later in Chapter Ten.

VII

Profit vs. Nonprofit Communities

You cannot judge the quality of care you will receive based on an establishment's charitable or for-profit status. Keep in mind that many large corporate entities target profit margins of 30 to 35 percent. If you are paying five thousand dollars per month in a 30-percent profit margin scenario, $1,500 of that goes to stockholders, owners, or investors. In contrast, if you choose a nonprofit, it could use that $1,500 in margin to start a new program or service inside the organization or to cover better benefits for employees. The bottom line is stewardship of resources.

While one might hope that for-profit or non-profit status would clearly delineate one thing or another, it does not. In generating targeted profit margins, organizations develop a culture whereby the operational expenditures are maximized to deliver the best product possible to compete well in the marketplace. This can also be true in non-profits where margins are committed to frequently upgrading the physical plant, providing additional services or staffing or putting away funds to support residents who have exhausted their financial resources. It is generally true in for profit communities that do not accept Medicaid, that once you have exhausted your financial means, you will have to leave the community. I have, however, known of for profit communities who extended discounts on fees to extend the length of stay. This is generally not the case with most large organizations that do not accept Medicaid or some other form of subsidy.

If the availability of indigent care such as Medicaid or subsidies from the organization is high on your list of desirability, ask these questions up front. "What happens if we run out of money?" One of the phenomenal product features of a life care contract is that it provides care for life. If funds are exhausted these communities often rely on Medicaid reimbursement in the nursing home environment or subsidies from a non-profit foundation to support the cost of continued care within the community. We will talk more about life care contracts and continuing care retirement communities in Chapter Ten.

Publicly traded companies provide access to their financial statements and conference calls for analysts and Wall-Street types. Nonprofit entities file tax returns that can be reviewed on GuideStar.com. Financial information about communities such as non-profit CCRC's receiving municipal bond financing can be found on www.emma.msrb.org. Ask for financial information you may want to consider in your decision-making process. Most non-profit organizations compile year end financials and make them available to interested parties. You can check for CCRC accreditation at www.carf.org. While accreditation indicates financial strength and some level of quality in the operation, there are excellent CCRCs who choose not to become accredited. Communities pay CARF a fee to receive accreditation.

Get a feel for the company by talking to the staff. Here are some questions you might ask:

- Is the company burning to be the largest senior living company in the country, gobbling up other companies and growing at a breakneck pace?

- Is the focus on the residents or just on getting *more* residents, a greater profit margin, and increased growth?

- What is the tenure of the local leadership, such as the department heads, the executive director, or the administrator? Who was the last director? Can you give that person a call for a reference on the company?

- If there have been four mergers in the past five years, are the billing systems, policies, procedures, and corporate services the same from community to community?

- Have the newly purchased properties been integrated into the parent company?

- Is the location you are considering an original property or newly acquired?

- Ask for references from family members whose loved ones have either expired or moved from the community.

When it comes down to it, organizations strongly mirror the values of their leadership. This is why you need to get to know the community. People make the product. Quality care is local. For-profit entities can lose focus on residents if their fervor for growth and profit eclipse their core business. Nonprofits can become inefficient and unwilling to advance with industry changes, retain poorly performing or ineffective leadership, and be overseen by community boards with differing visions and agendas for the organizational focus. A strong consideration is personal resources. Charitable corporations often provide a safety net such as Medicaid or philanthropic funding to care for a resident who exhausts their funds. Most for-profits give you some referral resources and a thirty-day notice to move out when you run out of money. Investigate your options and ask questions. People, not brands, provide care and love.

Generally, the most highly profit-driven organizations choose to locate their senior living communities in high-density areas that have age and income demographics to support their profit margins. With capital more readily available to a successful, for-profit entity, buildings may be more sophisticated in décor and more tricked out with bells and whistles, but don't be fooled. The steak is not the sizzle! I never saw a Queen Anne antique chair that could answer the emergency call system. Nor have I ever seen a front lobby bistro that could pour coffee and provide refreshments for residents without any staff.

More moderately priced or independent operators may choose less populated areas or their city of family origin in which to operate their business. They may have less capital available for state-of-the-art call systems, wallpaper, and fixtures. This does not mean that they do not provide good care. When you come to the major aspect of the senior living product, it is love, compassion, and concern for the happiness and well-being of residents. I have seen cutting-edge computer software for memory support never used. Staff was never trained on it. Computer screens were too small for residents with vision impairments to read. Computers were located in inaccessible or distant rooms and staff did not encourage residents to use the computers. There was poor lighting or ventilation in computer areas. In essence, it is not about the bells and whistles of what you have. It is about what you do to improve resident life with what you have.

Continuing care retirement communities that need multiple acres to build multiple levels of care may be located in suburban or developing areas where larger tracts of land are available. This can make for a beautiful, pastoral campus with acres and acres of green space. It can also be distant from medical services, retail shopping areas, and restaurants. Many offer life care contracts that secure your need for care even if financial resources have been exhausted.

Nonprofits, many of which serve the indigent or those with less financial resources, may focus their resources on care and staffing. This is not a bad thing. So evaluate the building for cleanliness, safety, and comfort first. Look at the bells and whistles last.

VIII

Lifestyle and Care

Authenticity: Walking the Talk

Many national providers and large nonprofit organizations promote "signature" components of their living experience such as fresh-cut flowers, herb gardening, family nights, and a variety of other great ideas. When these signatures are well executed and held closely as part of the mission of the organization, it is evident. I started in the industry as a sales and marketing professional, and let me say up front that there is no more compassionate, loving, or mission-driven group of people in any industry. Your sales representative can be your confidant, consultant, and friend. You can easily grow to love this person, who can provide a smooth transition from family stress to a lifestyle that can open a parent's life to a whole new dimension. If you cannot imagine this happening with your salesperson, either you may need a new one or this may not be the community for you!

Let's take gardening as an example of a signature service. A senior living brand may present gardening as a signature of the community. In advertisements, you often see lovely, fifty-something models reminiscent of Grace Kelly posing in their pearls with a gardening hat and tools. This is marketing. This is not always reality. Again, be pragmatic in your assessment. You may walk through lovely herb and flower gardens that smell heavenly and make you want to move in yourself. Put aside your emotions and think the situation through. Consider these questions if your mom or dad loves gardening and you consider this activity to be a primary satisfaction driver for your loved one:

- Is the activity organized on a regular basis and led by a paid staff person, or is it self-directed?

- Are gardening areas accessible at early morning and at other times of the day that are natural to your loved one?

- Does the emergency call system extend to the patio or outdoor area where the garden is located?

- How many residents are involved with gardening at this point? Can your sales representative name a few? This tells you how well staff and management know the residents and to what extent lifestyle after move-in is a priority of the team.

- Are planting beds at an accessible height for residents working from a wheelchair or assistive device? Gardening may be a beloved activity, but if the setup and structure of the program does not lend itself to accessibility, will it really improve life quality?

- Ask residents if they have heard of the gardening activity. Is it on the activity calendar? Do you see photographs and evidence of a commitment to the program in newsletters or photos in public areas?

Finally, if gardening is on the national website and no gardening is happening, this doesn't always mean foul play.

Residents have preferences. Gardening may have given way to pottery making, bridge, or a variety of other activities that are driven by resident interest and involvement. If a community is truly listening to its customers, there will be adjustments and responses to the offerings.

Life Example - I operated a community once where we provided lamb chops as part of the menu. Immediately after opening the community, a majority of residents voted lamb chops off the menu in our town hall meeting. "Nobody eats them." "Lamb is expensive. I'd rather have steak." "Stop wasting our money on something we don't like." There was near riotous disdain for lamb in the building! One year later, I heard someone ask in a resident council meeting, "Why do we never have lamb?" I looked around and assumed that everyone would explain that lamb had been voted down. Much to my surprise, we had had a good number of residents move in who were all lamb lovers. Things change. Maybe some of the other non-lamb voters were too quiet to express their love of lamb in earlier resident meetings and now were comfortable enough to vote for lamb. Who knows? We added the lamb back to the menu.

Great senior living communities love their residents enough to listen. When you have the right people in leadership positions, senior living is much like a family. We love macaroni and cheese, and then we graduate to junior high. Then we like hamburgers. And so on…

The bottom line is this: What you smell is what you get. What you see is what you get. Whether physical smells or *experiential* lifestyle activities, walking the talk creates evidence of the walk. Look for it.

Reason #3: I Don't Want to Live around Those "Old People!"

This is my personal favorite. It indicates that people consider themselves a part of a much younger and more vibrant group of human beings than those they perceive to live in retirement communities. They may be comparing themselves to residents of a nursing home or assisted living facility. It may or may not be a correct evaluation. The MacArthur Foundation Study on Aging in America (1998) found three key behaviors related to aging well. They are: (1) low risk of disease and disease-related disability, (2) high mental and physical function, and (3) active engagement with life.

In many cases, the retirees who present Reason #3 may be actively engaged with life. This is a good thing, but not a reason to eliminate exploration of senior living. These seniors may be involved in volunteer activities, dating, travel, or jobs. They see no reason to slow down and consider retirement living, nor do they think of living in these communities as desirable in any way. They choose their own friends. They make their own schedules and do as they please with no time for whining. In my experience, people with this personality profile will indeed live stronger and longer.

In some cases, they are absolutely right! It may be too soon to move to a retirement community. It is not, however, too soon for them to educate themselves on their future choices. Realize that the ability to engage in life changes as your situation changes. Retirement communities have evolved considerably in recent decades. Senior living communities are an excellent venue for retaining access to social networks, developing friendships with others in similar life situations, and maintaining involvement in activities that support high mental and physical functions. Make sure you get to know your options. Set aside time to have an intimate and compassionate dialogue about your family's plans and to hear each other's perspective and expectations.

Parents: Initiate the conversation

Your children don't want to think of your aging process. They certainly don't want you to think they are thinking about their inheritance and making the depressing assumption that you will not age well. No matter what stage you may be in in the decision-making process about your life plan, share your thoughts. If you would not be comfortable with family members providing personal care, explain this and communicate your plan. Many seniors today see planning for their needs as a gift to their children. Making the choice proactively for provision of care and services makes it more likely that the time you spend with family will be high quality time. Discussing laxatives and bodily functions is not a comfortable approach for some seniors. Your privacy and self-determination is your own to orchestrate. Communicating your planning and expectations is a healthy way to strengthen family bonds and avoid rough patches later when expectations might cause discord due to poor communication.

Children: Initiate the conversation if your parents don't

Express your respect for your parents' independence, security, and well-being. Reinforce that you want them to experience *choice* and *self-determination* as they age. Be honest about what support you can, and hope, to provide. If caring for your parents has always been your expectation, discuss the importance of this with them. Negotiate your need to be a good child with their desires for your involvement. Discuss your capacity to support their aging process within your own family unit before bringing it up with your parents. Communicate that you want to know and understand what is important to them. This is not a morbid endeavor, nor is it doom and gloom. If you take no other advice from this book, please consider these proactive recommendations carefully.

Document the conversation so that you will be informed and organized should decisions have to be made based on the information exchanged. Your family may be one of genetically gifted stock that does indeed live stronger and longer, with members expiring in their sleep at eighty-eight years old after a full day of shopping at the mall! What a blessing!

Questions to Consider

Do yourself a favor and imagine what you would want to know if it becomes necessary for your family to consider a senior living community. Below are some questions families should consider.

Lifestyle

- **What if certain activities I currently participate in are no longer a part of my life?** Would I need to consider moving to a retirement community? Many seniors who live in retirement communities continue to work full-time or work as consultants in areas from medicine to accounting. While this component should not be a determining factor, a loss of capacity for or interest in employment may indicate a need for a new socialization outlet or variety of activities that a community can provide.

- **Are there experiential programs I would enjoy?** Experiential programs provide access to new experiences and the learning of new skills or information. These are programs that provide life experiences such as travel, lifelong learning, and cultural pursuits. Does the community provide assisted travel? Day trips only? Weekend getaways? Cruises or trips of extended duration, such as seven- to fourteen-day excursions?

- **What kinds of educational opportunities, such as lifelong learning, are available?** Many communities provide on-site lifelong learning programs in cooperation with local universities. Some communities provide tiered access to local universities with transportation. Be careful to ask very specific questions. While private universities often have strong affiliations with either owned or affiliated retirement communities, public universities, which are funded by tax dollars, are limited in providing services beyond what your citizen peers can access. Be clear about the affiliation. Is it affiliated with an alumni association? The actual university? Or does the community provide access to public programming by providing transportation or support services? It could just be located near the university and that's it. Ask to see class schedules or speak to the resident leader of the program. Attend a class!

Care

- **What is included in wellness and exercise programming?** How many full-time employees does the wellness department employ? It is not surprising to find websites and brochures populated with multiple references to wellness. Investigate the offerings. Ask to see a class schedule. Is the exercise facility certified by the ICAA (International Council of Active Aging, www.icaa.cc)? Do the offerings match your (or your loved one's) interest level? Is there an indoor pool? Is it heated year-round? Are organized aquacize classes provided year-round? What are the certifications and specialties of the staff? Kinesiology? Physical therapy? Are classes tailored to all levels of ability? Assisted living? Memory care? Nursing care? As with dining quality, it is not uncommon to see specialized, sophisticated wellness offerings for independent living residents only to find that the offerings are different for other residents (e.g., the lifestyle coordinator may only teach chair exercise to the residents of assisted, nursing, or memory care areas). Comprehensive wellness programming becomes more important as people start to lose capacity and ability. Engagement in physical exercise can increase appetite, as well as maintain muscle mass, balance, and mobility. Physical activity helps to prevent depression and provides a sense of well-being and self-determination.

- **In this community, does wellness mean proactive health maintenance, or is the "wellness nurse" someone who deals with physical illness?** It is important to understand how language is used in a given community. For example, in many assisted living communities, a wellness nurse is someone who coordinates and oversees the medical care of a resident, *not* someone who oversees proactive wellness programming.

- **If personal or medical care is needed, is it provided as part of the community continuum of care, or will it be necessary to move to another building or another community when care is needed?** Considering the transition from one life stage to another can be a crucial factor. What types of care are provided? What conditions require a move to a higher level of care? Does this require moving to another building or area or will I have to leave this community and find another? If your resources are limited, you must consider what happens when they are depleted. Does this community accept Medicaid or have financial support programs to guarantee care for life? Is the care provided by the parent organization, or is this an independent living community with services for care contracted to other providers? If life care, what foundation or fund supports care for those who have exhausted resources? How is this fund replenished, and is there a qualification process to access this means of financial support?

IX

Parents Are People Too!

Dating and Relationship Considerations

For active, independent seniors, it is important to consider relationships and socialization. A parameter to consider is the availability of social and support networks. If Mom and Dad are located in a suburban area where driving is key to social choices, what are the markers to consider when friends or peers start to move to retirement communities or relocate to be nearer family as they age? Include important social relationships in the dialogue; whether intimate or platonic—people need people. This conversation will enhance a proactive awareness as the social network changes, diminishes, or relocates. A proactive approach may actually enhance the process, as friends may choose to investigate retirement options together or verbalize bonds that are important to maintain.

It is well to consider that the option of relocation, when choosing a retirement community, has a major impact on quality of life. While keeping parents and adult children nearby might give the child a sense of security and identity as being a "good child," it can also isolate and break the parents' close supportive ties to lifelong friends. While relocating Mom and Dad from Connecticut to California in a lovely retirement villa, purpose-built in your backyard, may give the child a sense of security and alleviate the guilt of geographic separation, it could well create separation and isolation from lifelong friends for the parent(s). The adult child may envision an idyllic family compound with Mom and Dad engaging with and watching their grandchild learn and grow. But the reality may be that a resentful teenaged grandchild must now clean up the mess left in the yard by his or her grandparents' ten-year-old Labrador, which is doing nothing to enhance the family relationships.

Adult children need to remember that their parents have lives, independent and autonomous from the adult child. I have had adult children show up to visit their parent at her new assisted living residence only to find that Mom is dating a new guy, and they have gone on an outing to lunch and gamble at the local casino. A wake-up call to say the least. Sensitivity and objectivity are important to the discussion on relationships. Our parents are adults. They don't always disclose their most intimate relationships and certainly feel no need to shatter our perceptions of their lives when it calls for disclosing details that illicit shock or dismay. Our ideas about lifestyle are certainly not always shared. Communication is the key to mapping out a plan that works on all fronts.

Exercise

After discussing priorities for aging well, compile separate lists of what you have heard and what your parents feel they have communicated as their satisfaction drivers for aging well.

- Identify life changes that will necessitate decisions.

- Discuss assets and financial limitations.

- Set a time to compare your lists.

- Align your priorities with theirs when your resources and lifestyle allow you to do so.

- Honestly communicate your limitations in meeting their expectations. Whether other family obligations, career, or geographic separation play a factor, analyze the feasibility of your involvement.

Map a strategy to identify what actions might be taken to react and improve lifestyle quality when:

- relationships and support network diminish

- functional capacity diminishes or interferes with preferred lifestyle

- geography, transportation, or other factors interfere with quality of life

Ask them to investigate options for reacting to changes. Investigate options such as living wills and medical and durable power of attorney. Identify decision makers when self-determination is no longer possible. Agree on how and to what level you can support them.

> *Reason #4: I'll Cross That Bridge When I Get to It. Gladys and I Have Each Other. We Don't Need a Retirement Community.*

While Gladys may be the most beautiful and graceful woman to ever live, she is not immortal. Keep in mind that she is also aging. While she loves you dearly, she probably doesn't want to end up changing your undergarments. Nor you hers! You have options. There is nothing inherent in taking care of oneself, and planning for our own aging needs that makes one any less compassionate, loving, or committed. If you truly love your partner, and he/she you, it is good to remember that your own aging is inevitable.

If you have each other, give yourself a hundred bonus points. For many people seventy and over, a significant loss of relationship may have already occurred. As we age, we lose people. This does not always mean a death of a spouse. Friends move to retirement destinations. Friends alter their lifestyles. Couples divorce or change partners, and socialization patterns are altered. People downsize to smaller homes, active adult communities, golf communities, and lake houses, often relocating to be nearer to their children.

Those exceptional, motivated, educated, and self-sufficient children you raised learn to speak Chinese and take your grandchildren to Hong Kong because Computer Worldwide recruited that exceptional child you raised. Celebrate! You did your job. A-plus work. After you celebrate, realize that your same capacity for delivering a phenomenal adult human being to the world can be focused on delivering another thirty years of a thriving life filled with joy and productivity. You worked for it. You earned the right.

Turn your attention to the life you and Gladys want for yourselves. And don't trail off and lose enthusiasm for your plans at eighty-plus years. Many seniors plan travel. Relocation. Dancing. Right up until they get to the life plan that covers eighty years old and beyond. The verve trails off, and either people joke that "I'll be dead by then!" or "We'll be over at Shady Acres!" You may not be at Shady Acres if it is full with a waiting list.

Don't under-plan and under-expect for the last semester of life. It can be one of the most enjoyable semesters! Remember cutting class during high school to go to "college day" at every community college and university in your state! Remember taking a road trip during school hours, unbeknownst to your parents, just to hang out for the day! Remember how the teachers almost gave up on keeping you focused and sitting in class. Truth be known, they were a bit tired too and knowingly gave you a little rope to start your adult life. Just like being a senior in high school, being a "senior" in life provides a waiting horizon. It is all in your attitude. Your kids aren't keeping you "in class" as a parent anymore.

While you and Gladys don't *need* a retirement community, make sure you drill down on life choices and clearly define what you *want*.

Do You Want...?

- **To maintain the home and the yard you needed earlier in life?** As we live longer, life costs money. Would you rather spend your assets on insurance, yard maintenance, and taxes or on some other life-enriching pursuit such as travel? When you consider that insurance on the average family home is going to run you $1,400 per year and that insurance on a 960-square-foot condo in Fort Lauderdale, Florida, built after 2006 to hurricane specifications, will be less than $400 per year in some cases, what will you do with your choices? I continue to mention that our generation is living stronger for longer. This impacts the magnitude of these decisions. While someone forty years ago might expect to live twelve years in retirement, you may live thirty. A thousand dollars of insurance saved per year saves you thirty thousand dollars over your retirement. It just got interesting, right?

- **Routine?** Routine is comfortable, but is it what you *want*? We love our bridge game on the cul-de-sac. We love our dry cleaner. We love Maria's Italian Restaurant, but we've had all that for thirty years. With so many choices, do we really want to spend another thirty years the same as the last thirty? Maria's will still be there when we stop by, but really, another thirty years of Maria's every weekend?

- **To be home base for your children?** Our children grew up here. We want them to have a place to come home to. Really, Gladys? You've given them eighteen years—sometimes thirty these days with the new generations X and Y. Their education and rearing has taken them to Hong Kong, and they Skype once a week. Is this a delusion that somehow you are responsible for being the rock of suburbia when your kids fly back to spend thirty-six hours in your home once every two years? I will certainly respect your right to live in denial, or on the Nile, but you have to decide in a moment of conscious reality. I won't allow you to tread water for the next thirty years without having had the conversation.

- **To sit around and wait?** For what? Your friends to move to Arizona? Your church Sunday school class to shrivel from thirty members to five? Your whole neighborhood to turn over so you need to wade through fifteen bicycles to get to your front door? All your friends to live life while you get the occasional postcard and sit through three hours of slides when they come back from Brazil? Your cousin to run away with a sixty-year-old Salsa instructor and buy a house in Belize?

If you want to sit and wait, just remember you could be waiting for thirty or even forty years. You may not realize it, but so many of those seniors you pass on the freeway that you consider to be in your peer group at seventy-five are actually ninety-three and on their way to doing something interesting. If nothing else, living in a community with a few ninety-plus-year-olds who are running circles around you might either motivate you with a new perspective or challenge you to give aging your best work and grow up to be just like them!

As I referenced earlier, living in senior living or a retirement community does not mean a nursing home. I cover the kinds of senior living communities next in Chapter Ten.

Denial: I'll Cross That Bridge When I Get to It

As with many significant life transitions, there is no one road map that works for everyone. With aging, the bridge comes to us. Either we will be prepared and cross it firmly in control of our own destiny, or it may be a bumpy ride all the way across. With this bridge, it may well be the last one we cross and have more significant and irreversible ramifications than the preceding ones. Is it any wonder people don't want to think about it?

Denial is not an advisable strategy and can lead to catastrophic outcomes. Temporary or crisis approaches to care and assistance can quickly deplete resources, leaving your family with no permanent life plan in place. Financial and familial outcomes that allow the bridge to overtake us can lead to the elimination of *choice* and *self-determination*.

Realize that Reason #4 is you giving up your choice and self-determination. In many cases, this reason might as well be "I'll let someone else take care of that." While this may seem like a comfortable way to remain in denial, consider the consequences. Relinquishing your self-determination while you have the capacity to make your own choices might not seem like such a big deal right now. As your capacity to take up the reins becomes diminished, however, you may regret missing the window of opportunity to take the reins at an appropriate time.

John D. Graham

Maintaining Health and Social Well-being

Research indicates that socialization and community are valid indicators for maintaining health and happiness as we age. Consider aging as an Olympic sport. Who does better? Athletes who train in their hometown with their hometown coach, or athletes who better locate themselves geographically, engage the expertise of new communities, seek competition, and socialize with other athletes who aspire to be Olympians? I would assume from the behavior of Olympic hopefuls that the latter is true. Aging is much the same way. Those who start conscious aging well earlier, those who learn in and with community, and those who are disciplined in the pursuit to live stronger and longer do just that.

As with any endeavor, focusing on the task at hand delivers increasing returns on outcomes. To approach aging with a "wait and see" or "wait until I need it" approach is shortsighted, to say the least. A sure way to relinquish *choice* and *self-determination* is to wait until a facilitating event dictates your choices. Absent information on the options and identification of a responsible party, someone will eventually make your decisions for you when you lose capacity. We all age, and with aging come health challenges. With health challenges comes the expenditure of resources. With the expenditure of resources, lack of resources can follow soon behind if not properly managed.

Just as long-term care premiums are affordable when we choose to purchase them at a younger, healthier age, there is a point after which investigating long-term care insurance becomes a waste of time. The window of opportunity has passed.

The same concept applies to aging. There are windows of opportunity at functional levels along the way to integrate exercise, intellectual stimulation, social engagement structures, meaningful work endeavors, or volunteer positions that may impact our ability to live strong. If we forego all the proactive steps we can take, it becomes time to hold on to our hats and checkbooks and ride the aging wave. Proactive, good aging is much the same scenario as securing insurance. As we lose capacity, our choices for care and services narrow, and guess what? The price goes up, both in well-being and actual financial outlay.

Life Example

<u>*Scenario #1*</u>

William, a healthy, seventy-six-year-old senior, might choose to invest $250,000 in a 90-percent refundable life care plan at a continuing care retirement community. At seventy-six, Will has some normal health considerations related to aging but still qualifies for a life care contract. This investment might allow him to leave the 90-percent refund of assets to his family and pay a stable, consistent monthly fee as he ages through assisted living or memory care. He may ultimately need skilled nursing on the same campus where he entered at the independent living level. Let's say he is paying three thousand dollars per month at the independent living level with meals, transportation, housekeeping, fitness membership, etc.

Will makes new friends who are living stronger for longer. In essence, this Olympic aging athlete has moved to Lake Arrowhead to work on his skating and keep himself strong in a community of like-minded others. His new friend, Elizabeth, asks him to go to the symphony with the gang, and Hal and Edward, his new Friday night poker buddies, invite him on a variety of day trips and golf outings to keep him in the game. He starts to work out with Hal three times a week to stay strong for golf. Will doesn't want to be the one who gets old first and can no longer play! Edward, a new friend, had a fall two years ago and takes balance classes. Will decides to go to balance class just to see what it is about and finds that it is a good way to keep the blood flowing after breakfast. It is really a good, well-paced class that seems to help his joints feel better, and the day just seems to flow better from the burst of energy he gets from the class. He also decides to take a class in European Renaissance architecture organized through the local university. It meets one night a week and is held on campus, so no night driving is required.

Scenario #2

A parallel option might be to forego the investment in a life care plan at seventy-six. In this scenario, Will remains in his own home and waits for the bridge to come to him. He's lived in the neighborhood thirty-five years and still has a friend, Ernest, who lives two blocks over. They meet occasionally at the local diner for Saturday morning breakfast. In waiting for the bridge and staying at home, Will does not engage in exercise or feel any peer pressure to age well. Instead of using his developed balance capacity to go on trips to the symphony on Thursday night or to enjoy local travel options, Will stays at home and starts to isolate himself a bit. He's not quite comfortable driving at night, but he still shops for groceries during the day, prepares his own meals, and occasionally plays a round of golf. So many friends have moved away or still have their spouses, and he really doesn't feel comfortable going to the symphony alone, although he and Barbara, his late wife, were season ticket holders for many years. He sees Sandra, the housekeeper, once a week, and he ends up watching a lot of TV and sleeping more than usual. The gardener comes once a week, but Will usually just waves through the window or interacts minimally for trimming instructions.

After three years of missing Barbara and living this less-than-optimal, scaled-down life, Will falls while stepping over the tub into the shower. He is in the hospital for three days and then checks in to a nursing home for rehabilitation for almost a month. It seems that his sedentary lifestyle for the last three years and a diet of peanut butter and crackers has not left him as strong as he used to be, and bouncing back is laborious.

After Will leaves the nursing home, Brad, his son, finds a nice woman, Tina, who comes for four hours a day and helps Will with his bath and chores around the house. Brad was hoping to get the shower *reworked so Will would have some bars to hold onto, or he was thinking about possibly even taking out the tub, but he had to fly back to Denver for work. Will is having some mild depression and low energy levels due to the pain medications working through his system, not to mention the fact that he needs to use a walker, which keeps dragging on the carpet. He knows he will get better eventually, but the therapist no longer comes out to work through his exercises with him, and progress seems to have stopped.*

Will passes the desk he used for so many years. He sees a pile of bills related to his hospitalization. Who can figure out Medicare? Bills for co-pays... Bills for caregivers... Bills for medications... Brad could help, but he is working seventy hours a week now. What to do? Mail this all to Brad? Who does he call to help him figure it all out? He needs to transfer money into checking to take care of the bills, but he just can't remember the access code. Will feels sad about the weakness he feels and the loss of his ability to walk. Will starts to feel very alone. He cannot drive. Even if he could, there's no one covered by insurance to take the car out to have the brakes replaced. It's just not high on the priority list right now.

Sandra has taken on more clients since the in-home caregiver came to help, and Will misses her company. Sandra had helped Will and Barb for over twenty years. The new caregiver, Tina, is nice, but Will is uncomfortable having her in the house so much, and they really have nothing in common.

With three kids, a thriving career in architecture, and Barb, the most beautiful girl in the world, who knew Will would end up living alone with Tina, his new life companion?

While this scenario seems bleak, I have intentionally not included all the details in coordinating care, home maintenance, transportation issues, Medicare coverage, and providing for activities of daily living. Countless hours have gone into allowing Will to come home. And to what? Curtains that remind him of Barb? A stranger in his private space with whom he has no relationship? Bills stacked on the desk? Peeling paint on the house and a neighborhood, once full of friends, where no one even stops in to say hello? While I could continue with this scenario and leave you grieving for Will's losses, I think you get the point. *"Waiting to cross that bridge when you come to it"* can leave you alone, feeling isolated and facing challenges on every side with little support. This scenario can also leave you with rapidly depleting assets and the need to either move from place to place to get care or to stay home alone and struggle to find care.

Comparison of Scenario #1 and #2

If we compare the scenarios, we can see that securing the life care contract does not prevent physical issues from happening. It won't bring Barb back. It won't move Brad closer to home. However, it does provide a plan and a support system where Will has professional staff to support all these transitions. It provides rehab care right on the campus where he lives. The social worker in the nursing home on campus helps to explain how Medicare and co-pays work. A pharmacy delivers all his medications and sends one bill at the end of the month. The life care service provides transportation wherever he needs to go. The apartment has an emergency call system with floors and a shower designed for aging residents. Meals are delivered. Care is provided without a stranger being in Will's home four hours per day.

Far more importantly, in Scenario #1 Elizabeth stops by every day to check on Will, both while he is in the nursing home for rehab and after he moves back to his independent living apartment. She picks up his dinner meal from the restaurant on campus, and they spend the evening watching some TV. Hal encourages Will to come down for the Friday night poker game two weeks after Will gets home. He has an emergency call pendant, and the hallways have handrails. Will uses the walker the first few weeks to get down to poker but finds, after a month, that he can make his own way down to poker, and he's even winning a few dollars! Will can feel himself getting stronger. Soon he will be back on the bus and heading to the symphony with Elizabeth.

Edward, who had a fall earlier, keeps encouraging Will to do more. He connects Will with the state senior health insurance volunteer who comes out and helps Will work through a problem he had with a bill. Edward is going gangbusters after falling two years ago, and Will knows he can bounce back as well.

Elizabeth is a wonderful person, and Will has started to bond with her great-grandson, Seth, who attends a local university and works at the fitness center on campus. Seth is getting his degree in kinesiology and assures Will that he can get his strength back. They start out slowly and work on balance, adding some light free-weights. Seth recommends a Pilates class using something called a Cadillac machine. Will starts making great progress. The machine allows him to strengthen his whole body and focus on the muscles used to support his upper body while learning to walk regularly again. His lower body still has some pain, but Edward assures him it will get better with time and hard work.

I hope this comparison will enlighten you to the idea that being proactive can make a significant impact on quality of life. Waiting for the bridge to come to you is, in essence, giving up and waiting for the challenges that come with aging to either overwhelm you or leave those around you burdened with a sense of guilt and uncertainty as to how they can help or what kind of help you need. The retirement years can be a wonderful, rewarding, and enjoyable time of life, but like anything else—career, sports, relationships—the aging process requires engagement and energy. Waiting for the bridge to pop up is about as smart as standing in the middle of the street and waiting for a car to come. If it is a street, eventually a car will come, but the middle of the street is no place to be. If you are a human being, aging and the challenges it presents will come. Being alone and uninformed is NOT where you want to be.

As a sidebar, I will offer some advice that is an old adage in the industry. You want to be the most needy resident in assisted living but the healthiest resident in a nursing home.

This means you get the most attention in an otherwise healthy group in assisted living. When it comes to nursing care, you want to be the healthiest, most cognitively intact resident to voice your needs and preferences. As functioning declines, choices such as when to bathe, when to eat, and when to drink can become more institutionalized and integrated into the convenience of the operation of the community rather than dependent on your personal preferences.

X
Senior Living Options

In order for you to exercise *choice* and *self-determination*, you need to make not only educated, but also timely decisions. Below I outline the different types of senior living choices as well as some in-home options. Choosing any of these options requires timely decision making.

Active Adult Communities

Active adult communities are limited to those fifty-five and over. These communities may be rental or ownership, with minimal monthly service fees that provide for some services such as housekeeping, meals, use of common areas, activities or outings, landscaping, and even home maintenance. They may provide swimming pools, fitness centers, catering for events, or travel/transportation services. Active adult communities target younger, active seniors. Waiting to move to one of these communities until you are eighty years old could be very disappointing. The activities, interests, and capabilities of residents will skew toward pursuits that require good physical capacity and endurance that may be beyond people in their later years.

Naturally Occurring Retirement Communities (NORCs)

Naturally occurring retirement communities (NORCs) may not be planned communities for retirees but are areas with attractive features for seniors where older people naturally relocate. These areas could include a new condo development downtown near the arts district with trendy, modern lofts, or a suburban, mixed-use development with condos located over retail and office spaces. These developments usually have an abundance of amenities such as shops, restaurants, fitness venues, and even businesses where you might walk right downstairs to your part-time job. They allow for integration into communities with multiple generations and sometimes offer cottage-type stand-alone units up to larger single-family homes on the perimeter away from the town center.

Should you choose a NORC for your retirement years, be aware that your plan also needs to include provision for possible frailty and care needs as you age. Due to the demand in these areas, you often find care resources serving other residents and thus accessible to you as needs arise. It is good to consider as well that limitations of the building may not bode well for needs you may develop as you age, such as large turning areas in baths, elevated appliances, and assistance with transporting groceries.

Section 202 Housing

These buildings are developed for the moderate-income senior. Started by HUD, they accept a reasonable percentage of your income as payment for occupancy. While these buildings are designed for independent living, some are starting to offer services such as a meal per day. Some have outside agencies that provide services to multiple occupants for activities of daily living such as bathing, grooming, dressing, and transportation.

See www.hud.gov for more detailed information on this option. Again, timeliness is crucial. Good HUD developments usually have a waiting list that can range from months to often years. Investigate now. Get on the list if you find the place you would like to be. LeadingAge (www.leadingage.org) can help you to locate HUD housing options in your state.

Independent or Assisted Living Rentals

While these rentals can be pricey, and not always necessary for the dollars expended, they are a perfect alternative if one of the partners is starting to experience some needs for care. They come in a range of choices and flavors, with services ranging from hospitality services such as meals, housekeeping, retail, and transportation to assisted living and memory care, where a full range of personal care is offered, right up to the nursing home level of care.

Independent living options are often a great option when one partner needs care, and you prefer to bring in outside agencies to do the care. Remember that rental options allow for the choice of flexibility. If life changes and you relocate to another community, there is usually only a minimal community fee or deposit to be lost. You avoid the lock-in of a real estate purchase or a life care or entrance-fee model community, where you may be locked in to the geographic location of the campus. Check out www.leadingage.org, www.alfa.org, or www.ncal.org to learn more about these options and their state-affiliated counterpart organizations. (See also Assisted Living in Chapter Twelve, Financial Considerations)

While not all of these communities have waiting lists, good ones often do. You may have a particular location in mind that is very desirable due to the aging demographics of the community. Make sure availability is reasonable within the timeframe of your decision-making process.

John D. Graham

Continuing Care Retirement Communities (CCRCs)

These communities can be corporate for-profit businesses. They can also be nonprofit, faith, fraternal, or university-affiliated communities that have community benefit as their motive rather than profit. There are a variety of products in this category, including life care contracts that guarantee you a full continuum of care for life for an initial investment, often called a buy-in or entrance fee. A life care community is always a CCRC but a CCRC is not always a community that offers life care contracts. CCRC's provide multiple levels of care that afford a resident the opportunity to age through the continuum. They may or may not provide life care contracts. Do not assume that a life care contract guarantees aging in place on the campus. Some life care contracts allow for services to be contracted with assisted living, memory care or nursing homes at another location. These levels of care may or may not be owned by the parent organization. You want to make sure what your contract provides.

The term buy-in can be misleading when choosing life care, because it indicates a purchase of real estate. Don't be confused. For most CCRCs, you are purchasing continuing care, not real estate. The communities allow you to live in residences to receive care levels from independent to nursing, but there is no actual transfer of real estate involved in the transaction. The amount of the entrance fee that is refundable ranges from one hundred percent at death or move out to zero percent. Generally, the higher the refundable amount, the higher the monthly service fees. The lower refundable scenario generally has lower monthly fees.

Entrance fee prices can also relate to the size of the independent living apartment. As care needs increase and one moves through the continuum of care, nursing and assisted living apartments are generally the same square footage for all residents. Consider the additional outlay for a higher entrance fee, when the value is only in independent living square footage. It does not translate to a larger apartment in care areas. Considering that your investment is ultimately in the care provided—not real estate—it is a given that choosing a smaller independent living apartment with a smaller entrance fee gives you the most bang for the buck. I have often seen single men, who have no concern for square footage in independent living, pay thirty, even forty percent less for their entrance fee receiving the same care when needed. Just a little tip for the smart shoppers out there!

Types of Life Care Contracts

Type A – is the most comprehensive life care contract providing for multiple levels of care. The entrance fee or "buy in" is generally the highest in this category. In return for your investment, residents are promised care for life through access to the increasing levels of care provided by the community. Monthly service fees may remain level over the course of advanced care with only yearly increases related to inflation or additional required services such as three meals per day (instead of one), medical supplies, pharmacy and other medical costs. Ask your community representative about additional costs that may be incurred when moving through the continuum. Type A contracts generally provide subsidies by the community or Medicaid options should residents exhaust their financial resources thus the term "life care". With increasing lifespan, this product provides a safety net for residents should they outlive their money. Most communities require residents to maintain Medicare co-insurance. As we discuss repeatedly here in the book, Medicare does NOT pay for long-term custodial nursing care. Medicare pays for short-term medical care services related to physicians, hospitalization and rehabilitation. Medicare is medical insurance NOT long-term care insurance. The unlimited nursing care provided through life care contracts may be an added benefit should Medicare determine that a resident is no longer qualified for nursing care or yearly Medicare benefits be used up. Life care provides for continued custodial care in the nursing area should it be necessary, after a Medicare covered stay in the nursing home.

It is generally true that if you have waited until you need assisted care to apply, you will not be accepted under a life care plan. Some communities do provide options for residents who are not accepted under the life care plan. This option is not the norm for life care communities, and while it does provide you access to multiple levels of care on one campus, Type A life care members take priority. So, for example, if you are a renter or covered under Type B or C contracts listed below and need a higher level of care, Type A life care residents' priority and apartment availability will determine whether they have the capacity to open this option to you on campus. If your contract provides for health services and no openings exist on the campus of the contracting CCRC, some contracts allow for the provision of this service to be provided at another location.

Note: In comparing products, "market (private pay)" monthly rates can exceed life care rates by 30 to 50 percent.

Type B – or modified contracts also provide access to housing, services and amenities in independent living but provide limited access to assisted living, memory care or nursing care. The contract may provide the resident with a benefit such as 90 days of nursing or assisted living care. After these allocations are used, residents may receive a discounted rate or may pay market rates. The options in this category are varied. In the interest of your peace of mind, I will not go into multiple scenarios under Type B. Your best strategy is to ask questions, document the answers and have legal counsel assess the benefits provided under a Type B contract. Long-term care insurance can serve to shore up your portfolio should you choose a contract that requires market rate payment for care services.

Type C - Fee for Service Contracts require payment of full market rate for care services. Access to healthcare is guaranteed but Type A or B resident access may take priority if also offered by the organization. Some communities do not require an entrance fee for a Type C contract and only charge a monthly service fee. State regulations vary but a Type C contract may be essentially the same as a rental contract with guaranteed access to healthcare services. While Type A and Type B contract independent living monthly service fees may qualify for the IRS medical deduction, Type C monthly service fees generally do not. IRS deductibility is based on the concept that some portion of care services are being paid for by your monthly service fee in advance of need. Essentially, a Type C contract is paid only for independent living monthly service fees and not subsidizing later care services expenditures so no portion is deductible.

Some communities do charge an entrance fee under Type C contracts which serves to subsidize the market rate paid when care services are needed. This allows for a discounted rate for care services. If the value of the entrance fee is fully used in this arrangement, residents may then have to pay full market rate for services needed.

Life Example

Life care contracts can provide tremendous value and security. If your family tends to have a long lifespan, your investment could pay off big. I knew a lovely retired school teacher who paid less than $50,000 for a life care contract in the 1980's. She had a modest pension income, assets from her home sale and some equity assets. She lived to be over one hundred years old!

Needless to say, she outlived her assets but needed nursing care for over twelve years. By the end of her life, the community had built a brand new state of the art nursing home. The market rate for nursing care was over $80,000 per year. She continued to draw her pension, with *the life care community subsidizing the additional cost of her care after her assets were exhausted. For a humble teacher, she lived like a queen from her wise investment. Some employees called her the "Queen of the community". She did hold court and bragged to everyone she knew how old she was and how long she had lived there. Many visitors thought she was bragging solely about the age she had reached. Many of us knew what she was really saying, "I made a smart choice and now I am laughing all the way to the bank with some of the best nursing care around at a bargain basement, monthly life care rate". Never underestimate the wisdom of a bit of age!!!*

Check out www.leadingage.org for more information on CCRCs and to locate state affiliate organizations. Good health at the time of purchase is a core component of this product. Prospective residents undergo thorough mental and physical assessments that determine their appropriateness for the initial independent living level of care. The CCRC model of care is based upon the ability of residents to maintain capacity at the independent living level for at least three to five years. Consider these independent monthly service fees as the premiums you pay for the benefits once care is needed. The fees paid by residents in independent living offset the higher costs of personal and medical care provided in the assisted living and nursing care areas of the campus.

In recent years, multiple models of senior living based on the CCRC model have evolved. Some communities actually do sell real estate that may be left to the estate and resold if the resident moves out or expires. These models do provide for the appreciation of an owned asset. Conversely, as we have seen in recent years, you risk depreciation and difficulty selling the unit. An owned unit must be sold to another age and income qualified resident approved by the community. Some communities must be paid a percentage of any appreciation and must approve the buyer. While the unit is being sold, any monthly fees must be paid by the family or estate.

Virtual CCRCs

Virtual CCRCs are a recent product development. With the real estate crash and corresponding inability of developers to garner the sales prices designed to allow the condos for life model to thrive, virtual CCRCs are becoming more and more popular. You live in your own home, apartment, or condo, and your service fees bring the services to you. This avoids the sale of real estate and corresponding higher threshold of entry into a residential community that allows for aging in place or multiple levels of care on one campus.

These communities are often owned by or linked to a CCRC that has actual campus facilities. The options may allow you to pay an entrance fee, pay monthly service fees, and access care or services as you need them. They can be provided in your home, condo, or other living situation and are generally less expensive in price. The lack of a physical living space and the corresponding costs of providing a residence allows for lower overhead and expenses. I am aware of virtual CCRCs operating in Michigan and other areas of the country. While not all virtual CCRCs require an entrance fee, the concept is generally similar. See www.leadingage.org to locate state Leading Age affiliates that may provide this service.

Condos for Life

This product was trending upward before the real estate crash of 2008. The two communities that I am familiar with are in San Francisco, CA and Bethesda, Maryland. This model is a very upscale, ownership model, with corresponding top-end prices. Residents purchase the condo generally with covenants imposed that require them to sell the condo to age and income qualified buyers who must be approved by the company. In addition to purchase costs, monthly fees can be substantial. The product allows a resident to access services in a true hospitality-driven model. For residents, services mirror a full service residential building, providing dining, concierge, travel, maintenance, and housekeeping services.

As personal or medical is needed, residents access services in their larger, more luxurious independent living residences allowing them to age in place. Care services may be provided by the sponsoring organization through home care agencies or with staff employed by the company. Some condos for life obtain assisted living licensure so that in-house staff may provide some level of needed services for an additional fee. Hospice services can be accessed for end of life care allowing a full continuum of care while living in one's own residence. Although this model has strong promise, it is currently designed for those with high financial net worth. The real estate crash and decreased home proceeds have taken a toll on the growth of this product.

Nursing Homes

Nursing homes are designed for the care of residents needing medical and twenty four hour nursing care oversight. Nursing homes accept private pay, long-term care insurance, and Medicaid reimbursement. Nursing homes often provide additional medical care such as rehabilitation therapy and memory care. Nursing homes are required to provide a physician as the medical director overseeing the programs and quality of care. You can learn more about nursing homes at www.leadingage.org and www.ahca.org. Leading Age membership consists primarily of a range of nonprofit senior care services. The American Health Care Association primarily represents for-profit providers. See additional information on nursing care in Chapter 13 – Regulation.

Group Homes

Group homes are sometimes called "board and care" homes. This model has been around for decades. For the price conscious, this can be a very affordable option. There are a variety of approaches, with some group homes even allowing seniors to live right in a family home with the family operating the business. The benefits can also be a corresponding disadvantage. Dining may be very much family style and warm, but choices can be limited. There is no restaurant. Caring relationships can develop between owners and residents with benefits to both parties. Residents pay a monthly rental fee for lodging combined with meals, housekeeping and personal care services.

Group homes exist for those with memory care and physical frailties. In recent years, we have started to see group homes with formal or informal marketing to affinity groups who share the same interests. Some examples might be all-male or female residences, veteran centers, or gay/lesbian/transgender-oriented group homes. Many group homes affiliate with the Assisted Living Federation of America (www.alfa.org) and their state affiliates. Some states have a large supply of group homes, and there is a separate state association representing these organizations.

Sorting Out Your Options

To start determining what kind of retirement community you may enjoy, there is a consumer quiz at www.retiringbydesign.com. Choose the "Resources" tab. Consider your desires in relation to the questions asked. This may give you a clearer picture of your choices. The questions can also serve as a springboard for family discussions about the appropriate level of care needed.

Senior Living at Home

With so many innovative approaches to living at home, a thorough investigation of these options is a must if your plan does not include senior living. With technology advancements, improved home modifications, and a variety of other developments, one can arrange for home care when needed. Keep in mind that this strategy must have a leader, someone to orchestrate the system of care. The staff has to be coordinated and often managed by you or your loved one.

The Potential for Financial Abuse

There are credentials to be checked for both agencies and individuals. You want to know that persons entering your home are ethical, law-abiding citizens. Inviting someone into your home provides possible access to financial records and valuables. With litigation at an all-time high, don't forget your liability if someone is injured or has an accident in the course of working in your home. One judgment can impact your nest egg tremendously.

Agencies generally check the backgrounds of employees they provide to work for you in your home. They usually provide drug testing results, criminal background checks, health screens, and previous employment verification. Know that people looking to evade the law or cause damage to you usually have a plan around these hurdles.

Life Example - I once employed a person who was so adept at building compassionate relationships with residents that she had no problem getting Uncle Ralph to write her a check directly. She gave dire accounts of her struggles to retain custody of her children and avoid the abuse of her wayward husband, as well as of her isolation from assistance from her family, who lived in another state. Financial abusers such as this woman are often sociopathic in makeup and don't have to directly steal anything.

This individual had a trail of financial abuse across the country, but she had never "stolen" anything.

When someone writes a check in sympathy, the verbal understanding may be that it is a loan or that services will be rendered in return for the money. Unfortunately, without a loan document, there is no evidence of the verbal agreement. One cannot be prosecuted for taking a gift from a senior.

Most senior living communities have a policy against any financial involvement between residents and staff. No tips. No loans. No gifts. Not even a soft drink from the fridge. Residents are often so grateful for the lovely caregivers they get to know that this policy can seem restrictive in allowing them to express their gratitude. Residents do ignore the policy. As we age and feel financially secure, our compassion for someone we care for and feel to be a good person can be abundant. Residents often think, "I am taken care of. I can never spend the assets I have. Why shouldn't I help this person with so many challenges and such low wages?"

While financial abuse can happen at home or in a senior living community, in a senior living community, responsibility for investigation, remedy, and recovery efforts lies with the senior living organization. You are responsible for filing the police report. So, while neither scenario (home or senior living) is perfect, there is value in having the systems and resources of a senior living organization to hopefully prevent, halt, or remedy these situations.

Caregiver Attendance

Caregivers are often the rocks of their own families. Demands from elderly relatives, adult children, and grandchildren can sap time and energy from the person who is of the caregiver mentality. Personal demands can interfere with their ability to show up to meet your needs. Agencies often attract workers who need the flexibility of part-time work or working when their personal situations allow. There is high turnover among workers. You may fall in love with one caregiver who chooses to work sporadically due to personal issues. There is also no guarantee that you will be assigned the same helper week to week or even day to day. Receiving a new caregiver leaves much of the burden on you for orientation to your home, expectations, and needs.

Turnover is high in senior care communities as well. It is common in the industry for the staff to turn over one hundred percent in a year. Turnover rates below fifty percent are very rare. So while senior living does not eliminate the work-force challenge, it does leave someone else responsible for managing it.

Twenty-Four-Hour Care

If your strategy is to stay at home until the end, consider that you may need twenty-four-hour care. This usually involves at least two workers or shifts per day, seven days per week. This is a staffing and scheduling challenge beyond the skill set of most individuals. Agencies work diligently to keep your time frames covered, but as you can imagine, it is challenging.

You have to consider who will have the time and energy to manage the staffing if you decide to age in place at your home. With your life plan, you may set up predetermined thresholds at which you are no longer comfortable staying home. For example, you may decide that when you need four or more hours of care per day, you will move to a senior living community. Be sure to plan the next stage. Decide:

- Which community?

- What is the time frame for admission?

- Do they have a waitlist?

- Should I put down a deposit to be included on the formal waitlist and contacted when openings are available?

Home Modifications

As your mobility declines, your home may need modifications such as grab bars, zero threshold showers, ramps, or other safety measures. The National Association of Home Builders (www.nahb.org) has a certification program for home modification professionals. Correct installation by a qualified construction company is important.

Grab bars generally have to have blocking in the walls to anchor the installation. Zero threshold showers must have skilled shower installers to get the floor angles correct so that water flows to the drain and doesn't end up on the floor to create a slip-and-fall incident. There are now perimeter drains that provide submerged drainage channels with caged covers that allow the shower floor to remain level while draining the surface area. Make sure that you engage someone with the proper skills and training to do it right. Think ahead and have your entire home done in one project if possible. Dealing with dirt, dust, and construction debris while you are not feeling well is not the preferred experience. If you have an injury such as a fracture, occupational therapists are generally a good resource for planning your modification.

Explore Your Options Sooner Rather Than Later

With all the options covered here, don't let fear be a stumbling block to exploring your choices before you *need* them. Depending on your spouse or family to study your choices—unless negotiated, planned, and agreed upon—can be a stressful mistake. Family members can have overwhelming responsibilities in day-to-day life with work, responsibility for children, financial pressures, and multiple aging family members.

Bear in mind that a couple in their forties or early fifties may have two parents each, four grandparents each, and possibly two remaining great grandparents well into their nineties. One family could have fourteen aging family members who have some expectation of support or care. This does not include aunts or uncles. While your family may be willing and supportive, aging happens for all of us, and it just may not be possible for them to support multiple family members adequately. Do you want to be the last one who needs help and is last on the list?

While we don't like to think about losing a spouse, you could be the one remaining. We have covered the scenarios with your spouse present. Consider your own transition after your loss. Living in a community with your peers, many of whom have experienced similar losses, can be a tremendous support. How many people in your current social network are eighty years old and dealing with the loss of a spouse after fifty years? It is a challenging time of transition, and you may want to consider the value of being around others who understand where you are in life.

I have seen multiple couples make the transition to senior living only to lose one or the other. When speaking with those who have been through this, I hear gratitude expressed by seniors for the love and support of their peers who have experienced the same situation: "I don't know how I could have gone through all our things and downsized after forty years in the house without my husband." "We would not have had such a clear financial plan and have our legal documents taken care of had we not handled this together." "I have new friends and neighbors to lean on who have been through the same thing." The words of gratitude are endless.

XI
Incorrect Assumptions Steal Your Potential

While no two individuals are alike, it is true that we gravitate toward people with interests similar to ours. Relationships are more important for seniors than at any other stage in life. Given the emotional transitions that come with aging, to be isolated without the opportunity for intimate, genuine relationships could be one of the most detrimental impediments to a quality retirement. It is good for us now to consider the importance of communities with interests and lifestyles we value.

Reason #5: I Don't Like Bingo!

While many seniors still love to play bingo, it is less and less prevalent these days in retirement communities. You most often see it in communities where the average age of residents is eighty or above. Bingo has really come and gone in communities more oriented toward the independent living resident.

Several hot trends in activities for retirees have emerged since the heyday of bingo. For several years, Wall Street rooms were popular. These were common areas designed for residents who wanted to use computers and fax machines, watch trading metrics on screens, and bond around money management. Everyone thought all the seniors were moving in with pockets packed with money, and their profiles suggested they were all CNBC addicts, day trading and compounding their millions. We all know this is not the case, but the perceptions were reinforced to some extent by news stories about "little old ladies" starting investment clubs and cashing in on the market. I know of few Wall Street rooms that remain. Seniors have their own computers and fax machines, and CNBC is available in your own apartment. While this may seem like a silly trend in hindsight, it does indicate the responsiveness of the senior living industry. As a whole, the industry is evolving into one of progressive ideas and a strong interest in serving residents' needs and interests.

Another activity that has lost popularity is bridge. Ten years ago, you might have seen multiple groups of bridge clubs with beginning to high skill-level players organized to play multiple times per week. You might see fewer bridge clubs today.

Woodworking, pottery, water aerobics, line dancing, sports, wellness, spiritual growth, and intellectual pursuits such as life-long learning classes are some organized activities that you continue to see. Senior Olympics have been around as a group activity for many years. Some compete in athletics at national levels and enjoy this venue of engagement immensely. Others think the idea of Senior Olympics is condescending and prefer to run a marathon without any age classification attached to their participation. Opinions on senior living activity are as varied as opinions on natural childbirth. People are people.

Progressive organizations are moving toward "experiential lifestyle activities." In recent years, activity coordinators have been renamed "lifestyle coordinators" or "recreation and lifestyle managers." This is evidence of a trend for the coming boomer generation to "experience" life rather than fill it with recurring "activity." Prior generations tended to focus on one sport or recreational pursuit, pursue that intently with a large amount of their free time, and often become focused on one area of recreation. Currently, we see economic trends that indicate our coming generation is less committed to locking in to one pursuit, whether that be tennis, golf, or skiing. The downtrend from golf, tennis, and country clubs to monthly membership yoga studios, retail spas, and dance lessons gives us an indication that we want to experience a variety of downtime choices; hence the term "experiential activities or programs." Another indication of the desire for experiential activities is the number of residents opting for assisted day travel groups who choose a variety of destinations.

Upscale communities offer services from memberships in local golf clubs to overseas travel to limousine transportation for a girls' night out. Consumers have and will continue to dictate to the marketplace when it comes to offerings. Their power and economic influence is no different inside a retirement community. If twenty percent of residents want regular transportation to the symphony, local theater, or health food markets, chances are good the company will respond and please its customers. If, on the other hand, you tour a community and see bingo on the calendar four times a month and no one there, or you see happy hour advertised at 4:00 p.m. and the bar vacant, you might question that establishment's responsiveness to customer demands. One of the great advantages of senior living is that your customer feedback can be instant, and in most cases, you can vote with your dollars and walk if you don't like the community.

Affinity Groups

Senior living communities also provide a platform to create affinity groups with your peers who enjoy the same things you do. When touring communities, meet multiple residents to discover interests represented in the community. Communities located near universities often have retired faculty and staff living there. They share the interest of similar cultures and work experiences. .

Some communities are affiliated with religious denominations or veteran groups. Air Force Village West in Riverside, California, caters to retired military. Areas around San Diego, San Antonio, and locales where military bases exist (or once did) may be populated with veterans. The community does not have to have a military branch in the name to gravitate toward retired military.

Sometimes locations attract a naturally occurring group of residents who chose to return to a community where they lived during enjoyable periods of life. For example, communities located near corporate headquarters attract residents who may have traveled with the company or been assigned to various company locations, but returned to retire in their city of origin. Rabid alumni from great universities such as LSU, Harvard, or Penn State migrate back to their college locales with plans for enjoying sports teams or taking classes. Those who love architecture, food, and the arts may migrate to New Orleans, San Francisco, or Chicago.

Location

Geographic locations can often give you a great clue as to whom you will find in the retirement communities in the area. It can be very rewarding to meet other people who have your same interests or values and have the freedom to enjoy retirement. Here are some examples of specific locations that attract retirees with specific interests or from certain backgrounds:

- Communities in **Florida** have a large number of residents who originated in New York, New Jersey, or other East Coast cities. If you love New York and big-city life, from delis to Broadway shows, your interests may lead you to Florida. If you retired as an executive from a publicly traded New York-based corporation, chances are you will find someone who shares your interests in major metro areas in Florida such as Palm Beach, Miami, or Tampa/Saint Petersburg. A great corned beef sandwich may not mean much to you now, but having one on the menu at age eighty might be a nice treat!

- **Arizona** is populated with "snow birds" from the Midwest who often fled the climate as active adults (ages fifty-plus). They fell in love with Arizona as active adults and possibly moved into retirement communities rather than returning to the Midwest.

- **Fort Lauderdale, Florida, and Palm Springs, California,** attract active gay and lesbian adults seeking community and decreased cost of living. Ultimately, increasing the LGBT population of senior living communities in these areas.

Finally, consider the location of family and friends. While you may have twenty family members living in the city where you currently reside, your assessment and future plan may not indicate that any of them are key factors in your care or lifestyle. It may be comforting to have them located locally, but don't have unrealistic expectations about how often they will visit or how involved they will be in care coordination if you ever need it. If you see them once a year now and you have to go to their homes for visits, chances are they are not going to be on your doorstep multiple times per year during your retirement!

Children, nieces and nephews, and younger family members tend to be mobile in their location these days. Younger people follow their careers or interests and may relocate five or six times before settling in one area. Communicate with your family about your hopes and see how they match your future plans. I am not saying that family will desert you, but chances are they have never really thought much about the ways they might be involved in your retirement years. Don't plan your future based on a faulty premise.

By the same token, adult children should not make assumptions about continuing involvement in their parents' lives either. Don't assume your parents want you to take care of them. Seniors are independent, often private people who shudder to think of their adult children being involved in their care. I have heard hundreds of residents who have chosen life care communities communicate that not being a burden on their children was one of their top ten reasons for choosing a life care community. Boomers, more so than other generations, have resources and added years to spend their resources. Their plans for successful life may be spending their last dollar on their last day.

If there are expectations or unspoken assumptions about inheritances tied to coordination of care, please have the conversation. Document your wishes and be clear as to what is expected of your heirs in exchange for inclusion in the will. I don't wish to be morbid, but it would amaze and probably nauseate you to know how many marginally involved family members expect their marginal involvement to be rewarded. As the relatives of these would-be heirs become frail and nearer the end, contact becomes more frequent, and interest in finances and legal documents escalates. I have seen the pattern over and over.

Life Example - Niece Jenny has promised to take care of Uncle Mark in expectation of an inheritance. She calls a few times a year, but Cousin Janice is picking up prescriptions, visiting at the hospital, and getting Fluffy groomed with no expectation of anything in return. Niece Jenny comes for a one-hour visit every two years and takes Uncle Mark out to the Sizzler for lunch. Jenny appears five times in ten years, but when Uncle Mark needs hospice care and is at the end of his life, Janice takes family medical leave and stays over until he passes away. If you are Uncle Mark, please make sure that expectations are clearly documented and upheld by the family member who agrees to care for you. Legal counsel can be appointed to draft these agreements and to make changes for you when expectations are not met. Again, walking the talk. Love is about the walk, not the talk.

In summary of this topic, as varied as it has been, senior living for our age group is not about bingo anymore. If your top reason for not considering senior living is "I don't like bingo," be aware that the phrase is a bit hackneyed and may pigeonhole you as exactly the behind-the-times, non-hipster you seek to avoid! People who think retirement communities are still about bingo are behind the curve.

XII
Financial Considerations

Reason #6: I Can't Afford It!

You may not be able to afford what you think you would like to have, but you cannot afford not to think about the future. We have discussed some affordable options such as Section 202 HUD Housing, virtual CCRCs, and freeing up fixed assets such as a large home. You know what your resources are, and you have to think about how they can best be used to maximize your quality of life. Think about it now. You may not feel like it or have the memory or capacity to make a good decision later.

Long-Term Care Insurance

Long-term care insurance can be purchased to secure financing of care when needed. It is also a wise strategy to preserve assets for a surviving spouse should one spouse need care and pass away first. I strongly encourage those fifty and older to consider purchasing long-term care insurance as a safety net to avoid depleting your retirement nest egg. It can also provide you with peace of mind in your early retirement years to enjoy the funds you have accumulated for more life enriching experiences than health care. Saving all your money for long term care you may never need can impact your ability to enjoy your active senior years.

Policies are available that provide a daily reimbursement for expenditures both at home and in a senior living community. Make sure that your policy provides for both options. The cost of premiums depends on your age and health status at date of purchase and the amount of reimbursement provided by the policy when you activate it. Policies can be purchased for specified daily reimbursement amounts, inflation riders to accommodate increasing costs of care and covered time periods from one year to ten. Naturally, the higher daily reimbursement and the longer your coverage period, the higher your premium will be. Some companies provide discounted rates for couples and even added discounts for couples sharing one benefit amount. Couples might purchase a ten year coverage period that can be shared between the two or used only by one spouse.

Gender also impacts the cost of your premium. With longer life expectancies and corresponding probability of using care benefits, single women pay higher premiums.

It is wise to investigate and secure long-term care insurance while you are healthy. Options include policies that pay a fixed amount per day for a fixed period of years, with a rider for inflation. For example, you might choose a policy that pays $150 per day for three years of coverage. For a single male the premium might run about $2200 per year and for a single woman about $3000 per year.

To qualify for benefit payouts, an individual must demonstrate need for the prescribed level of care. For example, some policies kick in when you need assistance with two or more ADL's (activities of daily living) such as bathing, grooming, dressing, housekeeping or medication assistance. Make sure to ask questions about reimbursement. Will the company pay you monthly in a qualified situation? Must you submit receipts for expenditures? What kinds of care qualify you to receive benefits?

Long-term care insurance can be a viable option for securing a quality aging experience. After many years of expanding options and increased competition in the product, some companies are dropping out of the long-term care insurance business. For many years, premiums were reasonably priced even for those well into their sixties, and many took advantage of this great window of opportunity. As life-spans continued to increase, many companies paid out more for services than they had predicted. They were not expecting so many people to live so long with care needs.

Plans can offer great flexibility in either receiving care at home or care within a residential community that provides personal and/or medical care. While receiving care at home sounds like the preferred option, (and you want the choice), remember that managing the care, the household, the bookkeeping, other medical insurance coverage, doctor visits, and a host of other chores are not done by the long-term care insurance company. You, your geriatric care manager, or some appointed individual has to manage the process. The company only reimburses you. See www.aaltci.org, the website of the American Association for Long-Term Care Insurance for more information.

Assisted Living Care

Assisted living can range from base rates of $2000 to $5000 per month in smaller cities with low cost of living rates, to base rates from $5000 to $8000 in larger urban areas. Multiple factors impact the base rate including size of the apartment, services included in the base rate, provision of memory care, cost of land and quality of the building and care. In addition to the base rate, assisted living communities often assess for levels of care charges as residents need more services. Assistance with bathing, grooming dressing, toileting, medication assistance and assistance with transfer or transport can all impact the charges association with higher levels of care.

When investigating assisted living, ask for the assessment criteria that will require you to move to a higher, more costly level of care. To levy a higher fee, most states require that responsible parties sign an addendum to the original contract agreement for the additional charges. Ask for copies of any agreements that might need to be executed at additional costs such as levels of care charges, medication assistance charges, memory care services and supplies such as incontinence products. You can expect cost of living increases to your charges yearly. These generally range from three to five percent yearly. Budget accordingly.

Medicaid

While no one wants to end up penniless and dependent on state or federal resources, it could happen if you live in denial. I am often frustrated when I hear about families investigating ways to divest their parents of assets and qualify for Medicaid-funded senior care. Transferring assets to family members in order to qualify for Medicaid services can be illegal. To consider breaking the law, one would think the outcome would at least provide a benefit worth the risk. If you rob a bank, you would hope you get away with enough cash to abscond to Mexico and lie on the beach for the rest of your life. If you are the senior in discussion, please know that divesting yourself of your assets, giving them to a family member who has no legal responsibility to care for you, breaking the law, and thinking life is going to be a beach may be the most faulty premise of all.

Medicaid-funded nursing homes are the primary resource for indigent care. *Medicare does not pay for long-term care in a nursing home.* Medicare is a health care program for medical care, not long-term residential care. In some states, Medicaid pays for limited housing options such as assisted living or community-based options such as day care. I know of no state that provides these more desirable, community-based services without a waiting list. While Medicaid nursing care may be more readily available, qualifying for it is no cakewalk. While you are allowed to own your home, your other financial resources have to be depleted to qualify, and you are usually given a meager personal living allowance of twenty to forty dollars per month. While the nursing home provides total care, think about what you ordinarily spend on magazines, shampoo, snacks, and other basic life expectations. Trust me: it costs more than forty dollars per month.

I am not saying that Medicaid-funded nursing homes do not provide good care. There are many organizations whose missions include providing quality indigent care. They are some of the most loving and laudable institutions you will ever encounter, but living in one is probably not going to be your first choice. With increasing health care costs and oppressive regulation, nursing homes struggle to provide quality care on meager state reimbursements. Most charitable organizations that manage indigent care subsidize the operational costs with private donations.

Let me give you a reality check. Private companies that provide Medicaid nursing care as part of their product offerings can generally afford to spend about five dollars per day on raw food costs for the entire day. What do you think? Can you currently spend five dollars per day on groceries to prepare breakfast, lunch, and dinner and enjoy mealtime?

The average cost of a private room in a nursing home is about $248 per day. Quality nursing home care in most urban areas of the country, with a population of 300,000 people or more, costs $7,000 to $12,000 per month. As an example, Medicaid may reimburse $170 per day, or $5,270 per month, for your care in a large urban area. This is reimbursement toward the top end of the range. Some states provide as little as $110 per day. Knowing that quality care costs between $7,000 and $12,000, do you think organizations can afford to provide high quality care on such meager reimbursements? If we use an average market rate of $10,000 per month, the disparity between the market rate of $10,000 per month and reimbursement of $5,270 is $4,730.

While nursing care is so meagerly reimbursed, the industry is the second most-regulated industry in this country. For anyone who has been involved in government oversight or regulation to any extent, please know that nursing care regulation is beyond what you can imagine. For several years, there was a trend in nursing care away from institutional models and away from using physical restraints to keep residents from falling. This trend is slowly reversing itself. With family litigation and regulatory fines for resident falls, many nursing homes have again started to restrain people in their chairs or put a whole floor of residents in a circle at the nurses' station so they can be watched for safety. If you are thinking of giving your money away to your family and breaking the law to get one over on the government and get five-star care for free, think again. Start sitting in a circle with your friends, watching a clock under fluorescent lights eight hours a day. That's your beach in Mexico!

With Medicaid expenditures rising due to the increased elderly population, federal and state governments are limiting expansion of the nursing home industry. You have read the papers. You have heard the numbers. Millions upon millions of seniors are aging every day, and there will be limited expansion of nursing care. Nursing home care is the most expensive to provide out of all the senior living options even considered for reimbursement. As I mentioned, Medicaid-assisted living and community-based programs are practically unavailable with limited openings. Government is quickly moving to find ways to discourage nursing care options and shift their burden for caring for the elderly through Medicare (medical care) and

Medicaid (long-term care) to health insurance companies in the private sector.

The federal government has collected your taxes for all your working life, indicating that it will somehow provide you with medical care under Medicare or indigent long-term care under Medicaid should you need it. In essence, the government has had an agreement with you. You pay taxes for this promised service, and the government will provide it. Now that we are approaching time for all these taxpayers to cash in their chips for these services, the government is looking to shift its responsibility to private insurance companies. In a nutshell, the feds are looking to maintain or decrease nursing home availability and shift programs to lower-cost, home- and community-based care services that don't involve costs for the housing portion, as nursing homes do. "That is all well and good," you say. "I own my own home. I want to stay home anyway. That suits me fine." This, however, is just an interim step in the overall strategy.

In the short term, home- and community-based reimbursement can be the humane, personal, preferred way to care for seniors. After this transition is near completion and everyone understands that nursing care will not be available for most on Medicaid, the big switch will come along. It involves the following argument: big government, Democratic or Republican, is no good at healthcare, so we are going to pay private insurance companies, who are the experts, to provide your care. Sounds reasonable. I think we can certainly get some agreement that government is not the most efficient in the area of health care. You will get quite a few seniors on that bandwagon. With that transition accomplished, the government will contract with private insurance companies to provide the care they promised. The care for which they collected taxes. The care provided will be far less comprehensive than citizens expect. The feds will pay insurance companies a capitated rate per month to take care of the elderly with some limited but monitored base levels of care, and voilà—you get what you get! Then, politicians can say it's just those bad-guy, capitalist insurance companies who won't give you the care you need. It's their fault. It is one of the great disappointments of history. You heard it while it was happening. Ringside seat. This, of course, is my opinion about the trends I see happening today. No one can predict the future.

PACE (Program of All-Inclusive Care for Elderly)

Home- and community-based (nonresidential, non-institutional) care options include day care, respite care—relief services so family members can get a break—homemaker services, housekeeping, transportation, and a variety of other services in different states. The most promising alternative that exists today is the Program of All-Inclusive Care for the Elderly (PACE). PACE uses a medical home model in which membership in a day care center or medical clinic is the central clearinghouse for all inclusive services. You continue to live at home, thus eliminating the cost to the government for the housing or brick-and-mortar component of long-term care.

The government combines Medicare (medical coverage) and Medicaid (long-term care services) reimbursement payments to provide one combined payment to a PACE provider to manage both care components.

Let's use an example of $5,500 per month. Medicare might pay $3,000 per month for medical coverage combined with a payment of $2,500 per month for the Medicaid long-term care portion from the state Medicaid program. Generally, the Medicaid portion is going to be less generous than the $5,270 payment for long-term care nursing services we used in our earlier example thus saving government outlay. Providers are paid one payment to provide or contract with other providers for medical care such as clinic visits, day care, physical therapy, psychiatric care, in-home support, transportation, transitional coaching after a hospital stay, home health, and other services.

The concept is that one provider is paid a capitated (capped) monthly fee to provide everything and anything that keeps you living at home and out of a nursing home.

The example is often used that if you have a dog prone to fleas, the fleas bite you and cause a medical condition requiring a hospital stay. The PACE provider can use these funds to exterminate the flea problem. In essence, PACE can provide any service, if the provider is willing to do so, that prevents the need for higher, more expensive levels of care. This comprehensive approach to holistic care is the most promising idea the feds have had in years. Suffice it to say, the hurdles in becoming a PACE care provider have limited large numbers of organizations from entering this arena. I have heard of applications for PACE provider status in the realm of two thousand-page submissions, with some providers working on the process for more than a year. You can locate PACE sites in your state at www.npaonline.org, the website of the National PACE Association.

While this holistic approach to care seems to be an area we should be moving toward, there are currently only a small number of PACE centers in the country, even though the program has been available for twenty years. Few organizations have the range of services required in place before developing the program. Some states such as Arizona do not allow PACE sites. In some states, you must have a medical clinic license and some depth and infrastructure to provide the basic services PACE requires. There is also the risk of catastrophic care to the provider organization. If you provide coverage to someone who cannot be maintained in his or her own private residence, costs can skyrocket, with only the basic monthly payment rendered to cover hospital stays and possible placement in a nursing home at the end of the person's life.

While the PACE model sounds promising, it does require that some portion of those seniors covered by a PACE center have care needs that cost well below what reimbursement is paying the provider to subsidize the higher care costs of others. All PACE enrollees must have health conditions that cause them to be nursing home eligible. So, to enroll enough healthier, stronger seniors who need fewer and less costly services within this nursing home eligible group can be challenging.

Medicare HMOs are paid under a similar capitated system to cover Medicare-eligible seniors. These HMOs want to keep the healthy individuals who cost less money and who will disenroll and return to traditional Medicare as they become frail or their needs increase. As a consumer, you may notice that younger, healthier seniors are targeted as enrollees by being offered free gym memberships and other generous benefits that might appeal to them. The HMO provider is aware that as seniors need more universal access to health care services, they may opt to move back to traditional Medicare coverage. This allows the HMO to make the profit on the lower-care senior while that individual is younger and less costly to insure.

This same dynamic would seem to be applicable to PACE programs. PACE programs need a mix of healthier nursing home eligible seniors. The value lies in the coordination and centralized access to care.

Keep in mind that PACE is currently targeted at the indigent senior—those who qualify for both Medicare and Medicaid. However, the concept also shows great promise for the senior with assets and a willingness to pay for care. Imagine the person who may choose residential care for the convenience of centralized and coordinated care who is willing to pay $5,500 per month out of pocket. If Medicare were to allow the private payment from the consumer to be combined with a capitated check from Medicare to the provider, this could be a great product. Many seniors own their own homes but have no family to coordinate the overwhelming amount of work it takes to coordinate care. This is not to mention the knowledge it takes to get all this done. The development of PACE for private-pay individuals would be a great comprehensive solution to care needs that would allow seniors the choice to stay home. You can learn more about PACE and how to advocate for expanded PACE services at www.npaonline.org.

Tracking Your Expenses

As you start spending money for personal or medical care, make sure you account for items for tax purposes. The cost of care, or, in some cases, the current expenditure for secured future care, such as life care monthly service fees in independent living, may be deducted as a medical expense on your federal income taxes. While your independent living service fees mainly cover housekeeping, meals, transportation, and other hospitality services, a portion is allocated, through actuarial computations, to finance your future care.

If you become a member of a CCRC community, their financial department will send you a year-end statement indicating that a portion of your monthly fees may be counted as a down payment on the future care you will receive in the community. My experience is that the portion recommended by your community may range from 0 percent to 15 percent, depending on the operations of the community. The percentage is just a suggestion. How daring you choose to be with the IRS is a decision you and your accountant must make!

Monthly services fees in assisted living, memory care, or nursing care are much more highly deductible, given that a larger portion of your fee goes toward the actual care of residents. A bigger chunk of your fee goes toward nursing staff salaries, upkeep of a medically designed building with emergency call systems, and specialized equipment and other medical specialty services needed to provide comprehensive medical care.

The Bottom Line

My detail here is not designed to discourage you, but rather to encourage you to plan and get yourself educated on what you can afford to allocate to the *care* part of long-term care. Exploring and securing your payment strategy for the care portion of your retirement can leave you with peace of mind to spend some of what you have accumulated to enjoy yourself—the lifestyle portion of your retirement.

You may think you cannot afford it now, but once you start to need care, the assets you do have can quickly be eaten up by poor choices, lack of information, and poor strategy. "I can't afford it" is denial. No one can afford everything, but you need to know what options are available to you.

As we have discussed care options, we have talked about Medicare and Medicare HMOs, which are the sources of medical coverage. We have also talked about long-term care—personal care combined with some ongoing medical care in a residential or home-based setting. Long-term care is paid for by the private assets of the individual, long-term care insurance, subsidized by Veterans Benefits or Medicaid, the state program for indigent seniors. Let's talk a bit about oversight of the quality and provision of these services.

XIII

Regulation

Each state generally has two agencies that provide primary oversight for senior living operations. The Department of Social Services or its equivalent and the Department of Health and Hospitals or its equivalent are the primary agencies. You will see the terms "health", "human services," "human resources," and a variety of other names used to name these agencies, but generally one is more oriented toward the social and daily living needs of seniors, and one is oriented toward healthcare-licensed settings such as nursing homes. Some states assign assisted living oversight to one or both of these departments, providing two different versions of assisted living and regulated by two different state departments. Senior living is also regulated by a variety of additional agencies such as fire safety, Department of Labor, OSHA, and the Department of Public Health.

Regulation of Assisted Living

Generally, assisted living has been seen as a "social model," with support services to assist residents with activities of daily living (ADLs) and not medical care. The assisted living industry started its expansion in the late seventies and eighties in response to consumer backlash against the institutionalization of nursing home care. As we mentioned, it's a very highly regulated industry. Regulation ensures some foundational level of quality in care. It also takes resources from operators in order to comply with regulatory hoops and generally leads to fewer choices for the consumer. On the good side, it shuts down greedy or careless operators who provide substandard or dangerous care.

Since the early eighties, assisted living has seen drastic growth. Consumers who did not want the regulated, routinized life in nursing care and who had the resources decided they would pay for their own care and get what they wanted via assisted living care. Regulators grew along the curve with the industry. Assisted living regulatory origins generally go back to "board and care" homes or a social model of living for seniors in a more independent or smaller home setting. Board and care homes were generally less regulated, with a lower need level by their residents, and thus assisted living has often been regulated under the assumption that it is really just a larger version of board and care. While this was true in the beginning, we have seen great change in the last three decades.

As assisted living grew, regulatory creep expanded to cover it. Consumers fled the "regulated, institutional" choice of nursing care to assisted living. Sadly, the assisted living industry continues to garner more and more oversight, with some states moving regulatory duties to the Departments of Health and Hospitals and away from Departments of Social Services over the past several years.

As we can see from the evolution of assisted living, consumer demand plays a huge role in product offerings. Initially, assisted living provided a more home-like residential setting than did nursing homes, and consumers paid out of pocket for the product. We discussed earlier that a very, very small percentage of Medicaid funds go to reimburse assisted living. As consumers demanded to stay in assisted living longer, the need for more medical care became evident. Assistance with medication, memory care needs, and other ongoing, but not terminal, care needs grew in the assisted living industry. Some providers started with one nurse, often called a wellness nurse, who was a licensed practical or licensed vocational nurse.

In the beginning, the primary responsibility of wellness nurses was to oversee medication reminders, assessments for needs for increased personal or medical care and on-site monitoring and coordination of doctor's orders. Consumers continued to demand that they be allowed to live longer and longer in nonmedical models of care. (Fair Housing regulations and, in some states, the Resident's Bill of Rights, allow for resident self-determination.) Thus, the senior consumer has expanded the industry to allow for new levels of care. Many assisted living communities now provide for increased care services, allowing residents to live in their communities until they pass away. The community will often assist with the coordination of home health care visits (medical care); oversight of care needs related to terminal illnesses such as kidney dialysis, chemotherapy, and radiation; and end-of-life care through hospice services.

As consumers have demanded more oversight, regulation has increased. Unfortunately, there are always a few bad apples among care providers and as complexity of care increases with our frail elderly, it is only prudent for us to make sure the care is being undertaken correctly.

Regulation of Nursing Homes

Nursing homes are regulated at both the state and federal levels. Nursing homes provide medical care overseen by a medical director who is a physician. Twenty four hour nursing care is provided on site, often with licensed vocational nurses providing the majority of care. Nursing homes can provide many medical services not available in assisted living. They can administer medications and do injections. They can provide rehabilitation therapy and wound care as well as expertise in oversight and treatment of complex medical conditions. Your physician can advise you when your condition requires nursing home care.

Many nursing homes provide Medicare covered skilled nursing or rehabilitation services related to a hospitalization and thus must comply with federal regulations to receive reimbursement. To clarify again, Medicare provides nursing care in response to a condition that requires hospitalization. It does not reimburse for ongoing, long-term custodial nursing care. Long-term nursing care is paid for by long-term care insurance, out-of-pocket funds or Medicaid for the indigent. Veterans are also entitled to certain benefits from their service in the armed forces. You can view star ratings to compare the quality of nursing homes in your area at www.medicare.gov. You will also be able to determine the number of nursing hours provided by each facility you are comparing. This site has a wealth of information on nursing care and regulatory issues.

State departments generally survey nursing homes once per year and state regulations vary from state to state. The agency charged with regulation can vary from state to state but generally have names that give you a clue. Some examples are Department of Health and Hospitals and the Department of Public Health. You can locate the agency charged with this responsibility in your state by asking your local nursing home or doing a web search.

Ombudsman Programs

Ombudsman programs provide advocates for senior living residents. They are often volunteers who are specially trained to investigate complaints from residents and advocate on their behalf. You can learn more about this program at www.ltcombudsman.org.

Regulation of CCRC's

CCRCs provide assisted living and nursing care so they are appropriately regulated by those state entities covering that particular specialty. In addition, most states have CCRC regulations administered by departments of insurance, financial services, aging or elder services or social services that oversee the entire community. Again, state regulatory names vary state to state. Two states, Alaska and Wyoming, have no CCRCs. Some states have minimal or no regulation.

CARF, while not a regulatory agency, is a national organization that surveys and provides accreditation to qualifying CCRCs. They examine financial performance, operational procedures and a host of other quality measures to determine if a CCRC receives accreditation. The process is requested by the CCRC and is completely voluntary. CARF accreditation provides insight to the consumer on the quality of the organization. (www.carf.org)

Also of interest, is a consumer association of CCRC resident members, the National Association of Continuing Care Residents Association. (www.naccra.com)

Regulation of Condos for Life

Even with regulatory oversight creep, the consumer continues to drive the product offerings. The "condos for life" concept that we mentioned earlier is a response to consumers who, in essence, just want the government to butt out of their care. Condos for life allow one to age in place, bring in the services he or she needs, and avoid assisted living or nursing-level regulatory oversight in some cases.

Most condos for life are considered independent living for regulatory purposes. Your personal medical services are not regulated in conjunction with living in the building unless they are licensed as assisted living. You are free to bring in the home health agency of your choice for medical care or for physical, occupational, or speech therapy. You are also free to bring in hospice care, nurse practitioners, or other services you feel appropriate. While these providers are regulated, they operate in condos for life as if you were in your own private residence. In essence, you get to live in your large, independent living condo without having to downsize to a regulated, medical care area. The hospitality services in these areas are generally more sophisticated and higher quality than one could access in nursing care.

My company, LifeSwell, provides support, education and assistance in evaluating options you are considering. I can be contacted at LifeSwell50@gmail.com or (818) 578-8917.

XIV

Stereotypes May Isolate You

> **Reason #7: Real Men Don't Live in Those Places.**

In the past, it was not uncommon to see senior living communities populated with over 90 percent female residents. Times are changing, my friend. Men are living stronger, longer, and in larger numbers. Men have tended not to live in senior communities. Women are more verbal, often more social, and seek the socialization a senior living community can provide.

Whatever your definition of a "real man," let me give you some ideas of how some real men have made the choice. We often hear arguments about enjoying keeping up the house, mowing the lawn, and working on projects such as auto repair, woodworking, and other traditionally male-dominated pursuits. While there are some holdovers from our past and more agrarian culture, today's macho man may be lord of the castle over an eight-thousand-square-foot suburban lot rather than a hundred-acre farm. Men have played the role of lord of the manor and traditionally, see themselves as the provider, caretaker, and leader of the family. The only problem with this is that an empty nest is not the same castle it was with a wife and three children to support.

Over the years, I have heard husbands voice their belief in the community living concept but relegate moving to a community to their wives after they have expired. Statistically, chances are you will expire first if you are male, but leaving the disposition of your belongings to your wife seems to me a self-serving approach. You leave your house and possessions of thirty years for your wife to sort through, discard as she chooses, and then pack up and move to a new environment once she has experienced the biggest loss of her life. For those guys who don't clean out the garage or the attic now and have tools they haven't touched since 1990, I guess this might be a pattern you are not going to break. Just give it some thought. If you haven't cleaned out the garage in twenty years, sorting it all out with your wife and moving to a community might be a life gift to make up for all the years she had to park in the driveway because the garage was too full!

Men who are truly motivated to give back their skills, wisdom, and leadership ability have found phenomenal ways to integrate their talents into a senior living lifestyle. If you consider the upbringing of today's twenty-something and thirty-something males, how many truly had the luxury of a fully present father? While your father may know how to patch sheetrock, replace a drain pipe, or install a lawn sprinkler system and may have taught you to do the same, the parents of today's young adults—with their harried schedules and faster lifestyles, soccer, debate team, and college preparation—have not always transferred those skills to the next generation. There are folks out there who need what you have to offer and would love to have someone with your wisdom and experience as a mentor and friend.

There are organized programs where seniors can give back, such as retired executives programs. There are community colleges where you can teach adult learning programs in everything from electrical wiring to masonry and horticulture. If your children have flown the nest and your grandchildren are geographically distant, trust me, there are people who would love to learn what you know and be happy to have your help. Whether the activities are organized or one-on-one, people need what you have to give, and living in a community can free you to share it. Programs such as Habitat for Humanity can allow you to contribute to the well-being of families and your larger community.

Loving the ladies? If you are eighty and still single and ready to mingle, there is no better place to find the company of lovely, available ladies. Senior living communities provide a relaxed, casual venue to meet datable partners who are generally polished, accomplished, and well-educated. The ratio of females to males is still easily four to one. There is a joke that I hear periodically about the available, single male senior: Two ladies are discussing the merits of the gentleman they are dating. One lady is raving over her latest beau. "Is he handsome?" her friend asks. "Does he have a full head of hair? Is he tall? Athletic? Rich? What makes him so great?" she quizzes. Her friend replies, "None of that!" She goes on to say that he has a car and he drives at night! For those of you guys who had challenges dating in your twenties, you may have some ideas that you don't want to go back to those days. Let me tell you, my friend, if you are eighty, have a car, and drive at night, your ship may have come in!

Relationships range from casual dating to intense, rapid courtships and marriage right on the senior living campus. Whether platonic or intimate, dating in your senior years can be a blast. Many people travel together. Take up a hobby or sport together. Go back to college. Map their family tree. There are all sorts of life interests that can bring people together for an enriched and enjoyable way of living that they might have thought long gone in their lives. Don't miss an opportunity in your last semester. Remember the high school example. Some guys who were gangly, awkward freshman grow up to be prom king in their eighties!

> *Reason #8: I'm Gay/Lesbian/Bisexual/Transgendered. I Wouldn't Fit in There.*

Don't be so sure. While our prior conversations about affinity groups, similar interests, and geographic preference hold true, don't be surprised to find older folks far more accepting than they might have been in their twenties. There is a mellowing and a wisdom that comes with age. Like fine wine, you improve with age. You live a few decades, and the world doesn't come to an end. You see a few economic depressions. Lose a few friends. And it seems that life lessons can give you a more measured approach. You learn that people are people. And that people who have lived lives differently than you have done OK. There are people you like and some you don't. People with whom you share similar backgrounds and interests and some you don't.

With time and years, people come to understand that rarely does one component of dissimilar lives disqualify you for friendship and camaraderie. I have seen some of the most conservative people have a few drinks at Mardi Gras with the least conservative and find similar interests, passions, and verve for life at eighty. I have been surprised to discover via demographic surveys that some communities you might assume were predominantly one thing or another are not. Choosing senior living is a behavior closely related to proactive behavior, education, income, and lifestyle. When you've been around the same kind of people for fifty years, sometimes you want to learn something new or hear about someone who has taken a different life path. It is that fabric of life that no longer threatens you, but enriches you. With many seniors being single and not looking for lifetime partnership, your sexual orientation is not as primary and differentiating as it might have been in earlier life.

Professional aging networks such as Leading Age, the nonprofit association of senior services providers, provide education for staff on gay/lesbian/bisexual/transgendered needs and preferences in senior living.

If you definitely would feel more comfortable with a larger percentage of similarly oriented individuals, again consider geography. Metropolitan areas with large gay populations tend to have more senior residents in communities of that persuasion. Areas such as San Francisco, Los Angeles, New York, Miami, and Chicago tend to have high gay concentrations. Gay retirement destinations such as Palm Springs and Fort Lauderdale tend to provide housing options where programming, activities, and socialization may mirror more closely the style of the general gay population outside retirement communities.

Options for the LGBT community are growing. Rainbow Vision Community was developed several years ago in Santa Fe, New Mexico. Oakmark Senior Living of Santa Rosa, California, has opened a lifestyle affinity community in Northern California. There are gay group homes in Fort Lauderdale. There is a Section 202 HUD Housing Community in West Hollywood that caters to gay residents. Desirable locales for gay people will continue to develop affinity communities as our population ages.

Meanwhile, don't rule out staying near your current location. If you have friends where you live now, encourage them to explore senior living communities with you. If your personal and professional life has been rich, rewarding, and full of meaningful friendships outside a senior living community, chances are, that will continue to be true if you move ten miles across town. I have seen gay couples live and thrive in senior living communities in the Deep South, which is often perceived as less comfortable for gay folks. It really comes down to individual relationships creating the fabric of a rich life. You will meet people with whom you enjoy spending time based on a broader spectrum of interests than sexual orientation.

As we age, there are some things that create bonds just by the nature of the years we have lived. Finding a good podiatrist may become a far more important factor than having a rainbow flag over the bar at your local watering hole. I was walking across campus one day and noticed a gay couple on their way to the fitness center to work out. To my surprise, they both had on shorts and black socks. Now, some of you may not get this, but wearing black socks with shorts is just something that most gay males *would not* do. It is, however, something most older males *would do*. I thought to myself, "Has the gay gene recessed and the senior gene become dominant?" What other explanation could there be for a stylish gay couple wearing black socks with shorts? In short, as we age, priorities change and people change.

Reason #9: I'm a Loner. I Don't Want to Be Around All Those People!

On the surface, this reason for avoiding senior living seems to be very reasonable, and it may well be if you are just a complete hermit. I have met very few people over the years who moved to senior living communities, namely CCRCs, who did not value the decision after moving there. When the individuals were independent and proactively made their own choices, the percentage of residents who report they feel they made the right decision and express happiness with CCRCs is in the high nineties.

I have encountered only three people in my career for whom senior living was just not the right choice. They should have stayed home or somewhere else. In one of these instances, the person just did not belong among the public, whether in a senior community, mall, or even a restaurant. Unfortunately, sometimes older people get a bad rap for being abrasive, demanding, or bossy. I have not found this to be true as a generalization. Mean people become older mean people. Nice people become older nice people. Mean people should probably stay home. Aging can present challenges to our mood. Aching joints, isolation, grieving the loss of friends, and life situations that would be stressful for anyone continue to be stressors. With any person, old or young, the more stressors you have, the more difficult it may be to cope.

So you are a loner! I can appreciate that. I am an introvert myself. Will I live in a senior living community one day? Absolutely! In addition to being a loner, I am also a frugal control-freak, and I want to make my own choices. A life care community where I can have support, assistance, and the dignity of choices will most likely be my choice. As a bargain shopper, I love a deal. For me, the idea of getting a locked-in flat rate (with additional meal charges as I move along in the continuum) at a CCRC is a deal I just cannot pass up. I plan to live a long, long time, and I love the idea of paying $3,000 a month for an upscale nursing home that costs the general public $12,000 dollars per month. It is just a deal that we coupon lovers cannot beat. It is a numbers game. You take the chance that you pay your entrance fee and don't live enough years to reap the benefit. I plan to get my money's worth and then some.

For loners, naturally socialization is not a primary reason to move to senior living. As with most people, the safety and security of care when you need it is the primary value of the product. Let's face it. If we never aged, senior living communities might not exist. I say might not, because there are empty-nesters for whom the socialization and peer encouragement factors are a huge value. They love the activity. The gossip. The scene. They want to be with the movers and shakers.

There is a certain component of community, even for loners, that is comforting. While you may not have thirty close friends or even know the neighbor two doors down, it can be nice to pass another human being in the hallway or have a chat one on one with someone sitting out under an oak tree. It is nice to have someone there when you are inclined to be sociable. Consider also that there will be other loners like you in the community. Some activities, such as life writing, book clubs, genealogy clubs, art classes, pottery, and historic preservation, attract those who tend to be more thoughtful and introverted. While the meeting portion is indeed communal, the pursuit of the activity happens when one is alone. Residents come together to discuss, learn about, or share the work they completed in private.

For those who prefer to be alone, consider making the decision to move to senior living as your needs increase. The socialization and community aspects may not be of particular value to you. Do not eliminate consideration of a CCRC if you have the financial means. The financial benefit alone may be well worth the choice. You may never need the care component, but the security of having care available to you and at a lower price point may well be worth the choice. You can choose to have meals delivered to your residence. You can choose to forego having the housekeeper come into your home. You can choose to never participate in a group or socialize in common areas, but the peace of mind and security may tip the scales in favor of some form of communal living. If not, you still must explore and decide upon alternative options. Whether you choose to bring care to your private residence through a virtual CCRC or to contract with outside agencies to provide care when needed, you must have a plan for aging well.

If you have a spouse who is a social butterfly, living in a community can be a benefit for both of you. Your spouse can go and be a social butterfly, leaving you to your own pursuits with no pressure to provide for the demanding social needs of your partner.

XV

Stuff, Stuff, and More Stuff...

It is indeed true that our generation in the United States has accumulated, owned, and used more stuff than any other civilization known to man. The advent of storage facilities on our urban landscape points to the fact that we have more stuff than we can even keep in our houses. What early twentieth-century citizen would have imagined that there would be a profitable industry devoted to allowing us to keep more stuff than we can use? I imagine the concept would have seemed as laughable to someone in the 1930s as a cell phone.

Don't let stuff interfere with your life! You can't take it with you, and, were you to be a fly on the wall after you are gone, you might be surprised at the value placed on your stuff. In one scenario, you might wish you had sold it and gone to Italy for several weeks because it was far more valuable than you imagined. In another scenario, you might discover that the item you think your heirs might squabble over ended up being sold for five dollars in an estate sale.

Reason #10: The Apartments Are Too Small! I Need Space for My Stuff!

Generally, you can categorize your stuff to see who needs to be responsible for it. If stuff makes you really, really happy and it is in your top five things needed to enjoy your life, I do not recommend that you get rid of your stuff, just so you can move to senior living. However, as we go back to our themes of *choice* and *self-determination*, we must ask who will make the decision about our stuff. Ask yourself:

- Why should it be someone else instead of me who decides what happens to my stuff?

- What will trigger me having to give up my stuff? If I have a health crisis, and someone else decides where my stuff ends up, how will that make me feel?

- How important is it that the stuff I specifically want someone special to have ultimately gets into his or her hands?

Part of the joy of accumulating and saving stuff is that magical moment when you give it to the person for whom you saved it. It is also important to stop and think about for whom you are really saving your stuff. Sometimes we think our adult children cherish their high school letter jacket or third grade art project when it is actually our grandchildren who would really be jazzed to see these things. These types of mementos provide a strong connection to their parents as young people. They help them connect with their parents. Having their parents' former belongings gives them a springboard to understand and have a history of details that might otherwise never be shared. An art project, a poem, a class picture, or a stuffed animal can be a cherished possession by the second generation. So, my purpose is not an argument for keeping or downsizing your stuff, but enjoying it in either case.

How to Categorize Your Stuff

1. ***Stuff you need/want to live now.*** This would be your stuff that you need or want to make yourself comfortable and functional for your life right now. If you like toast, then it's your toaster. If electronics are a big part of your stuff, list the stuff you use now. Not the word processor or the eight-pound mobile phone from your car in the eighties. Make sure you categorize your *now* stuff honestly. The 1,200-watt blow-dryer your daughter used for her seventies shag haircut may not be *now* stuff. Yes, she comes back to visit once a year, but she no longer has a shag, and blow-dryers are four times smaller now. Be realistic.

2. ***Stuff you think someone else wants.*** Before you address this issue, I have an exercise for you. Check out one of the great websites for estate sales, such as www.estatesales.net. Take a few Saturdays and experience several estate sales. Almost always, these sales are held after possessions have been distributed to family members after a loved one has expired. Visiting an estate sale need not be a morbid experience. If you like stuff, you might find something new! Just use it as an awareness exercise as you consider stuff you are keeping for someone else. After a few of these sales, you will realize that either no one really wanted this stuff *or* the person for whom the stuff was intended did not get it. Either scenario does make me a bit sad, but the bright spot is that your stuff can be better managed if you handle it now.

3. ***Stuff someone else DOES want.*** There are things that someone wants to have. This desire may have been

conveyed through conversation or may be an unspoken understanding. It may be the piano that you got for your son's lessons or a piece of jewelry that your only daughter will no doubt enjoy one day. Make sure you provide for orderly receipt of those items by those you want to have them. It is always good to consider when you should give the item away. Is this something you are using? Do you play piano? If not, this gift might provide your son's children with an opportunity to take lessons now. It could create joyful and current memories as you enjoy the piano anew while your grandchild learns to play.

Find ways to enjoy and create new memories with the items you are giving. For example, give one piece of jewelry to your daughter each time you have a special holiday dinner or occasion. Involve your granddaughter or great-grandchildren in hearing the history of the piece and the family story attached. Let the children tell the story on some occasion so they can remember the details for their children. Include several items in a memory box that you might pass along. For example, include the 1,200-watt blow-dryer, a picture of your daughter with the shag haircut, and an album of Carly Simon with the leather moccasins and bead necklace your daughter wore to her first concert.

Enjoy Your Stuff While You Have It

It is human that you have attachments to a life of possessions, so don't leave them in boxes. Let the joy of them come out into your life now. Share them. Discuss them. Keep them or give them away, but enjoy them. Don't let them sit in the attic somewhere and have the boxes opened by your heirs, who, in their grief and sadness, would give anything to know the story behind your things. Don't use your things as an excuse not to move on to the next phase of your life.

Identify all your stuff. The stuff that you or no else wants. Have an estate sale now, while you are here to enjoy it. Take the proceeds and do something you enjoy. Take the family on a cruise.

Downsize While You Are in Control

Considering senior living can be a process for many relevant life decisions in retirement. Many independent living residences have garages, walk-in closets, and even separate storage units that can be rented. So ultimately, stuff should not be the barrier that prevents you from moving to the next phase of life, should you choose. Your kids should not expect you to warehouse their lives like a museum for them to return to the shrine a few times a year. If they do, let them know times are changing and that you still have another thirty years to live. The less baggage, the lighter the load!

As you move to higher care levels in senior living, you will find invariably that the apartments are smaller. Assisted living apartments can range from 350-square-foot studios to scarce 2-bedroom units that might be as large as 900 square feet. Larger units are less available, and generally the percentage of 2-bedroom apartments is less than 20 percent of the mix of units. While assisted living apartments can have small kitchens, they are not equipped for cooking large meals. Nursing home units are generally much smaller. The norm is 150 to 250 square feet, and most have one closet and allow limited cooking.

As you consider your stuff around our theme of *choice* and *self-determination*, please know that downsizing while you are in control is generally far less painful. If you take the bull by the horns yourself, you may be downsizing from 2,200 square feet to 1,100. If you wait until you need assisted living or nursing care, the downsizing will be far more dramatic, and, chances are, you will be in far less control of the process. Usually a move to higher care levels is need-driven. At this point, you may have cognitive or physical impairments that drive your move. Others are generally making decisions for you about your stuff at this point.

XVI

The Final Pitch

As with everything in life, do what you do with vigor and wholeheartedness. If you are retired and have this wonderful life before you, choose what you will do. Be as determined in retirement as you have been in life up to this point. There are pros and cons with every life choice you make. Sit down and make a list of your possible options for enjoying life to the fullest. Narrow down the choices to the top five that inspire you with passion and energy. Some will be mutually exclusive. If you do this, then you cannot do that. Chances are, some choices involve a move, downsizing, or relocation.

Obviously, you cannot live in two places at once. Perhaps you have a primary home and a vacation home at the beach. If it has always been your dream to live at the beach, do it. Caring for two homes with insurance, taxes, utilities, and upkeep may only serve to slow you down. This is a prime example of why proactive decision-making can drastically improve the quality of your retirement life.

If your choices involve geography, narrow those down to your two most exciting choices. If you love your two-thousand-square-foot home, and owning it is your primary joy, focus on that. List the projects you always wanted to do, keeping in mind that adding a new bedroom for the kids may no longer be reasonable. Paint a room. Join a garden club. Take a course at your local university in interior design. Prioritize your housekeeping chores in a way that adds joy to your daily life. If you hate yard work, find a gardener who can take care of that chore so that you can focus on the interior. Make conscious choices. You were not given this abundance of added years in order to muddle through them as if you were home sick from work. This is a whole new life. Live it with passion.

As you think about the cons of possible locations, list things such as distance from friends and family, the aforementioned costs of maintaining your home, and security considerations. If you want to travel, there is an opportunity cost to weigh in this option.

You also have to consider your home as an asset. If your home is paid off, you should weigh the pros and cons of disposing of this major asset for cash. We don't generally live in our homes ready for a buyer. Interior furnishings can be dated or obsolete. When the market is hot and prices are up, chances are a buyer may be willing to overlook some of these obstacles. When the market is down, consider the time and energy that would be required to remodel, stage, and market your home in a buyer's market. The time and cash you may give up by remaining in your home could motivate you to make this decision sooner rather than later. Rest assured, selling in a buyer's market is a hill to climb.

Consider also the appreciation of this asset. If you paid $48,000 for your home in 1964, and it is worth $350,000 now in a hot market, is it worth the risk to wait? You could delay for 3 years and spend another $15,000 per year in costs to maintain the home. You could wait for 3 years and only get $300,000, with the possibility of having to pay for remodeling and staging costs at a later date. You could easily decrease the appreciated value of your home by $50,000 in 3 years. Meanwhile, you could take the profits, buy a smaller home, and get a return on the excess.

Remember, money has to work for you. Once you relinquish your career at the peak of your earning power, the options to return to your former earning power are limited. Consulting is an option, as is starting a new business or working as a greeter at a big-box store. But is that what you really want? Making your assets work for you instead of adding unnecessary cost is a key consideration in maintaining quality of life in retirement.

Hindsight is 100 percent accurate, but it is also irreversible. Time is money, and time is life. Whichever is more valuable to you, don't waste either. Live on purpose!

My mission with this book is to give you an overview of the reasons seniors avoid senior living. After considering these common objections, you may either have changed your reasoning or become more solidly convinced that senior living is not the choice for you. In either case, if your approach to successful aging has become more definitive or passionate, I feel rewarded. My prayer is that the information here has given you a springboard for careful consideration of the life yet to be lived. Family relationships are a cherished treasure. I hope this information can be a tool for nurturing and maintaining healthy family discussion as you age, a road map for living your best years yet!

A Message for Children

I pray this book has given you food for thought and some assurance that being there for your parents does not always end in crisis. While you cannot control issues such as denial, fear of aging, and resistance to change, you can be present and aware of the challenges. There is a saying along the lines of "What you do for others, God will do for you." Your participation and your concern for your parents' well-being will ultimately serve as a model for your children that will help them internalize the values of your family toward those who are aging.

In committing yourself to maximum *choice* and *self-determination* for your aging family members, you empower yourself with more preparation for your time in this stage of life. You create cherished moments that contribute to the fabric of family life. When the time comes, you are able to release your loved one, knowing that you both approached precious years of life with purpose and determination. After reading this book and sharing it with your parents, you are equipped with a springboard to start the communication process with your parents. A great future starts with the first step… a conversation with your parents. Make time for it and see how life unfolds!

Made in the USA
San Bernardino, CA
25 January 2016